Ultrasound Guidance in Regional Anaesthesia

Ultrasound Guidance in Regional Anaesthesia

Principles and Practical Implementation

SECOND EDITION

Peter Marhofer, MD
Professor of Anaesthesia and Intensive Care Medicine
Department of Anaesthesia, Intensive Care Medicine and Pain Therapy,
Medical University of Vienna,
Vienna, Austria

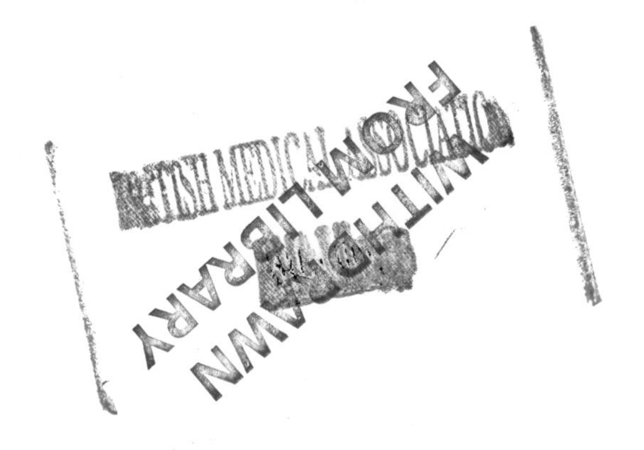

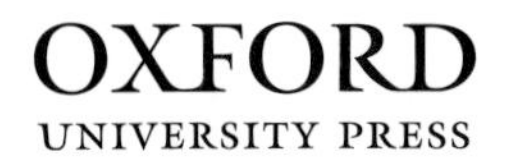

OXFORD
UNIVERSITY PRESS

Great Clarendon Street, Oxford OX2 6DP
Oxford University Press is a department of the University of Oxford.
It furthers the University's objective of excellence in research, scholarship,
and education by publishing worldwide in

Oxford New York

Auckland Cape Town Dar es Salaam Hong Kong Karachi
Kuala Lumpur Madrid Melbourne Mexico City Nairobi
New Delhi Shanghai Taipei Toronto

With offices in

Argentina Austria Brazil Chile Czech Republic France Greece
Guatemala Hungary Italy Japan Poland Portugal Singapore
South Korea Switzerland Thailand Turkey Ukraine Vietnam

Oxford is a registered trade mark of Oxford University Press
in the UK and in certain other countries

Published in the United States
by Oxford University Press Inc., New York

First edition published as Ultrasound Guidance for Nerve Blocks, 2008

Second edition published 2010

British Library Cataloguing in Publication Data
Data available

Library of Congress Cataloging in Publication Data
Data available

Typeset in Minion by Glyph International, Bangalore
Printed in Great Britain
on acid-free paper by
Ashford Colour Press Ltd., Gosport, Hampshire

ISBN 978–0–19–958735–3

10 9 8 7 6 5 4 3 2 1

Dedicated to my parents who supported me always

Contents

Acknowledgements

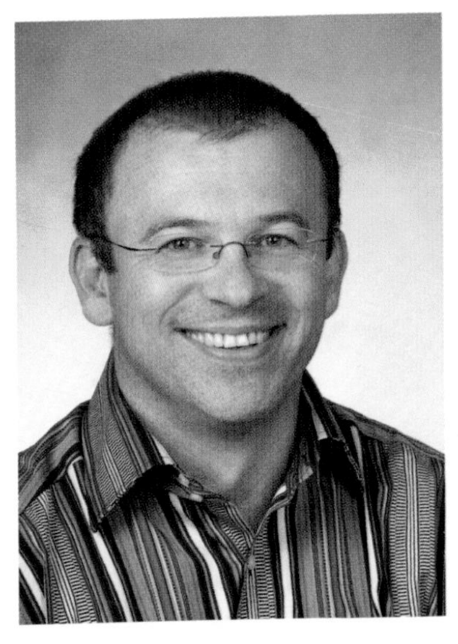

A book project like this can never be undertaken alone. Therefore, the author gratefully thanks:

Dr Lukas Kirchmair for his invaluable continuous cooperation, his excellent anatomy knowledge, the designing of anatomical cross-sectional images to perfectionism and proofreading of the entire manuscript. Thank you, Lukas!

Mitchell Kaplan for his excellent physics chapter. Even I understand ultrasound physics now. Thank you, Mitch!

Professor Bernhard Moriggl for patiently answering hundreds of anatomy questions over the past years. Thank you, Bernhard!

Professor Anette-Marie Machata and Professor Dr.Stephan Kettner for their excellent hand skills during the preparation of photographs. Thank you, Anette-Marie and Stephan!

Readers of the first edition for their constructive criticism.

Finally, all my colleagues who have been working with me for many years for resisting my (sometimes) crossness, and my wife, Daniela, for giving me the encouragement to complete such a project.

Foreword

Professor Admir Hadzic

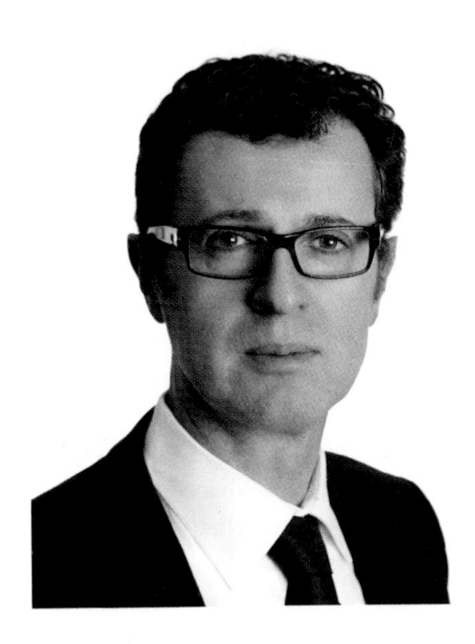

The practice of regional anaesthesia and peripheral nerve blocks in particular has changed substantially over the past decade. In fact, it would not be an overstatement to say that the new technical developments in the field tether of making some of the old teaching to the brink of obsolete. Most significant developments are the results of technical advances or, more specifically, the introduction of ultrasound monitoring for the placement of needles and catheters. The ability to monitor the disposition of the local anesthetic is now a key factor in acquiring an unprecedented control over technique execution. Ultrasound monitoring gives the practitioner insight into the block dynamics and disposition of the local anesthetics around peripheral nerves and plexuses. All of this new information has had a cumulative impact on our understanding of the mechanisms of neural blockade and the relationship between the volume of local anesthetics and a successful blockade. The idiosyncrasy of nerve stimulation, which was the gold standard for nerve localization prior to the introduction of ultrasound, is also much better understood.

However, ultrasound guidance during the administration of peripheral nerve blocks and increasingly, other regional anaesthesia techniques, was not an overnight success. Significant efforts were expended, both in advancing and improving on the ultrasound technology, to provide an image quality level that allows reliable imaging of the peripheral nerves and needle visualization. The industry clearly deserves accolades for their efforts to bring this technology within the reach of practising clinicians. However, these developments would not have been possible without the pioneering efforts of an international group of anaesthesiologists with extraordinary technical knowledge and drive. Indeed, it was the regional anaesthesiologists who fervently guided the industry to improve the equipment, and who then used every advance to test the applicability of the new technology for use in neural imaging and the administration of regional anaesthesia. It is for this reason that compendiums of knowledge from these very think tank echelons are particularly valuable. Professor Peter Marhofer and his Viennese group of collaborators are uniquely suited to create such a text. They have worked at the forefront to steer the ultrasound industry and the focus of clinical practice towards the application of ultrasound for use in regional anaesthesia since the mid-nineties.

This second edition of the well-received *Ultrasound Guidance in Regional Anaesthesia: Principles and Practical Implementation* expands on the first edition to include nearly all areas of clinical relevance. The second edition features some 200 photographs, including cross-sectional views of anatomy in human cadavers. A new chapter in this edition is 'Implications in children' which bridges the information gap on implementing the described technique in this population as well. Several useful appendices, such as expert consensus and the management of local anaesthetic toxicity, are also added.

Professor Marhofer and the contributors in Austria (Lukas Kirchmair, MD and Stephan Kettner, MD), bolstered by the engineering advice from Mitchell S. Kaplan, PhD, created a uniquely comprehensive, authoritative book on the use of ultrasound guidance in regional anaesthesia. The use of ultrasound guidance in regional anaesthesia has allowed for a myriad of modifications and variations of techniques, indications, and pharmacologic approaches, which inevitably vary from institution to institution. Not surprisingly, this volume represents the views and teaching methods of the fabled Viennese school. As leaders in the specialty of regional anaesthesia and the application of ultrasound, Professor Marhofer and the contributors compiled a uniquely outstanding and an authoritative text based on 16 years of clinical experience and decades of original research by the group. I wish to sincerely congratulate the authors and thank them for their immense contribution to the body of knowledge and pursuit of education in ultrasound-guided regional anaesthesia and beyond.

Admir Hadzic, MD
Professor of Clinical Anaesthesiology
College of Physicians and Surgeons, Columbia University,
Director of Regional Anaesthesia, St. Luke's-Roosevelt Hospital Centre,
New York, New York, USA

Foreword

Professor Narinder Rawal

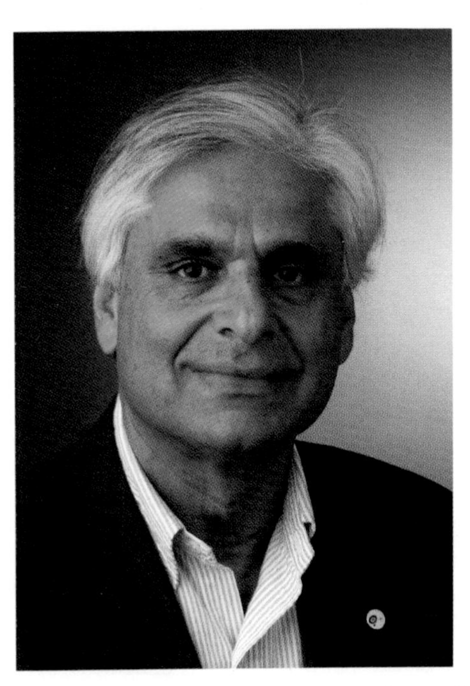

In recent decades, the role of regional anaesthesia has advanced significantly. Currently, it is widely practised for surgery in adults and children and also for the management of post-operative and labour pain. Improvements in nerve localization techniques such as nerve stimulation and ultrasound-guided blocks and the availability of stimulating catheters have improved needle and catheter placement. The accuracy and safety has evolved to such an extent that perineural catheter techniques are being increasingly used to treat post-operative pain at home after ambulatory surgery.

During the last decade, the explosion of interest in ultrasound visualization to guide local anaesthetic injection has been truly remarkable. Multiple national and international annual congresses, large numbers of dedicated ultrasound courses in various parts of the world, sold-out workshops at the European Society of Regional Anaesthesia and Pain Therapy (ESRA) annual and zonal meetings and other regional anaesthesia society congresses, the increasing number of publications on the topic, and the addition of a special section in the journal Regional Anaesthesia and Pain Medicine in 2007, all testify to the enormous increase in interest in ultrasonography in regional anaesthesia.

Ultrasonography allows the operator to visualize in real time the relevant anatomy, the nerve, the needle placement, and the spread of local anaesthetic. The enthusiasts claim that ultrasound-guided peripheral nerve blocks are safer because they have higher success rates and lower rates of complications, are non-invasive (as opposed to paraesthesia or nerve stimulation techniques), require reduced doses of local anaesthetics by about 30% or more, provide a faster onset and prolonged duration of blocks, and allow the detection of anatomical variations. However, there are others who are less impressed and have justifiably asked for good quality evidence to support these claims. This topic is a regular feature for 'pros and cons' debates in many congresses. There is a need for safety studies, efficacy studies, and equivalence studies of ultrasonic guidance versus conventional techniques for regional anaesthesia. In developing countries, the high cost of equipment is a major drawback. One may be for or against ultrasound-guided blocks and the jury is still out, but it is increasingly difficult to ignore the technique, especially in teaching institutions. It is also a generational issue that trainees everywhere seem to be asking for this technology. In short, ultrasonography in regional anaesthesia is here to stay and we can expect an increasing number of clinicians to practise this technique. Controlled studies to address the above issues can be expected to become gradually available which will establish the proper place of ultrasonography in regional anaesthesia in our armamentarium.

A good knowledge of sonoanatomy is crucial for a successful use of the technique. Acquiring technical skills is a major task and a correct needle-transducer alignment is the commonest error seen in the novices. This book by one of the pioneers in ultrasound in regional anaesthesia has now come out in its second edition. The first edition was published in September 2008 to critical acclaim. The author takes up the above issues of benefits and limitations of ultrasound-guided blocks. The 18 chapters also cover everything from the basic principles of ultrasonography and technical issues to blocks in different parts of the body, including neck, joint, and trunk blocks in addition to the obligatory upper and lower extremity blocks. In this second edition, Professor Marhofer has added new material which includes organizational and economic issues, paediatric applications, and the use of ultrasonography in neuraxial blocks. The overall quality of figures is better than in the first edition and cross-sectional anatomical illustrations are also included. There is a section on recommendations for the use of ultrasound-guided regional anaesthesia by a panel of experts from Europe, North America, and Japan. Professor Marhofer himself is one of the original experts with an experience extending to more than 15 years. His widespread experience in participating in ultrasound workshops in many parts of the world has been distilled into this new book.

In this book, every aspect of ultrasound-guided blocks has been covered in detail with emphasis on educating the reader for a safe and effective use of regional anaesthesia for surgery and pain management. This book will be a major source for trainees as well as experienced clinicians who will appreciate the wealth of information it provides for all practitioners of regional anaesthesia.

Professor Narinder Rawal MD, PhD, FRCA (Hons)
Department of Anaesthesiology and Intensive Care,
University Hospital Örebro,
Örebro, Sweden

Foreword: The surgeon's view

Professor Christian Fialka

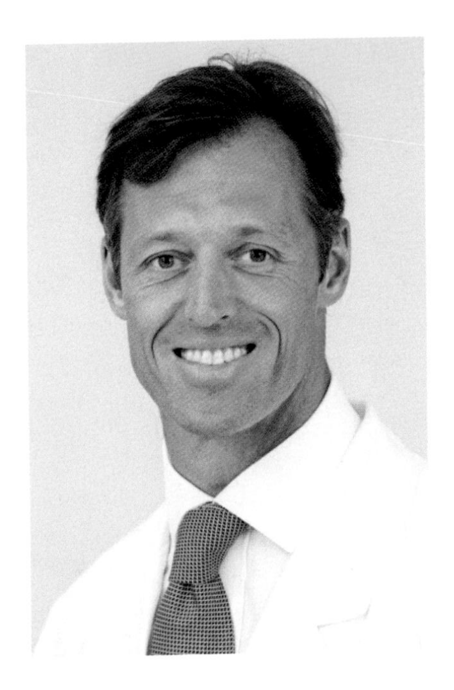

Regional anaesthesia in musculoskeletal surgery today represents the gold standard for a great variety of procedures. At our institution, we have the privilege to work with the group of anaesthetists who pioneered the field of ultrasound-guided regional anaesthesia, especially the senior author of this textbook. Therefore, over the years, it has become a safe and reliable method for almost all extremity surgical procedures.

In the early days, regional anaesthesia was not very popular in the surgical community. Neither landmark-guided nor electro-stimulation-guided techniques for regional anaesthesia could be used without showing a significant number of failures such as a delayed or incomplete effect and the need for an intraoperative conversion to general anaesthesia. Since we benefit from the development of the ultrasound-guided technique, the latter cases have become rare exceptions.

Other historical concerns such as the fear of delay due to prolonged preparation time before surgery, especially when compared to cases under general anaesthesia, disappeared during the past decade because of the positive experience from thousands of cases.

Today, ultrasound-guided regional anaesthesia is favoured not only during the time of surgery, but also because it provides a good post-operative pain care. For example, patients who are scheduled for arthroscopic shoulder procedures are provided with a single opiate administration subcutaneously (7.5mg Piritramid), 8 to 10 hours past the end of the procedure, using the rising analgesic effect of the opiate just before the block loses its effect and the pain level increases. Following this protocol, the amount of post-operative pain medication can be reduced significantly.

In summary, surgeons can recommend ultrasound-guided regional anaesthesia to all patients with standard procedures in bone and joint surgery. These patients are provided with a safe and reliable anaesthesia procedure as well as with a satisfying post-operative pain management.

Christian Fialka, MD
Professor of Trauma Surgery
Department of Trauma Surgery,
Medical University of Vienna,
Vienna, Austria

Contributors

Mitchell S. Kaplan, PhD
Principal Engineer, Advanced Development,
SonoSite Inc.,
Bothell, Washington, USA

Stephan Kettner, MD
Professor of Anaesthesia and Intensive Care Medicine
Department of Anaesthesia, Intensive Care Medicine and Pain Therapy,
Medical University of Vienna,
Vienna, Austria

Lukas Kirchmair, MD
Department of Anaesthesia and Intensive Care Medicine,
Medical University of Innsbruck,
Innsbruck, Austria

Bernhard Moriggl, MD, FIACA
Professor of Anatomy
Department of Anatomy, Histology and Embryology,
Medical University of Innsbruck,
Innsbruck, Austria

How to use this book

This book is written by physicians with 16 years' experience in ultrasound-guided regional anaesthesia. Focusing specifically on ultrasound-guided peripheral nerve block techniques, we avoided the inclusion of basic general knowledge in regional anaesthesia (e.g. indications and contraindications for specific blocks).

This second edition of the present book has been written after the great success of the first edition. The authors have carefully revised all chapters in order to provide the most recent knowledge in the topic of ultrasound in regional anaesthesia. A strong focus is still attached on anatomical descriptions and subsequent practical implementations. Paediatric applications are now included in this second edition in order to address paediatric anaesthesiologists too. Neuraxial techniques have also been incorporated to complete the entire topic.

We strongly suggest careful reading of the introductory chapters of the book. These include important information about physical background (e.g. how to adjust and fine-tune an ultrasound machine for optimal imaging), proven and potential advantages of ultrasound-guided blocks, and prerequisites for practical performance.

The chapters focusing specifically on blocks include precise descriptions about the relevant anatomy (including variations) for each block and guidelines for daily clinical practice in the operation room. Paediatric implications are added in each chapter where applicable. Essential information about each block is tabulated at the end of each description (see Table 1 for template).

Illustrated ultrasound images, corresponding cross sections, and the respective needle guidance technique are provided for each block description. Figures of the needle guidance techniques are shown without a sterile probe cover to demonstrate the exact position of the probe relative to the needle. Where useful, the position of the needle relative to the nerve(s) and/or the distribution of local anaesthetic are also included. All ultrasound illustrations are performed with SonoSite M-Turbo equipment except Figure 6.2, which is generously provided by Ultrasonix.

Table 1 Description of specific topics for each particular ultrasonographic-guided nerve block technique

Block characteristic	Basic, intermediate, or advanced technique (see Appendix 1)
Patient position	Typical position of the patient
Ultrasound equipment	Characteristic of the ultrasound probe
Specific ultrasound setting	Frequency of the ultrasound probe (high, medium, low)
Important anatomical structures	Description of adjacent anatomical structures (vessels, muscles, tendons, etc.)
Ultrasound appearance of the neuronal structures	Description of echogenicity and shape of the neuronal structures
Expected Vienna score	Visibility of the neuronal structures (see Appendix 2)
Needle equipment	Suggested length and tip of the needle
Technique	Description of the needle orientation relative to the ultrasound probe (**I**n **P**lane (IP) vs **O**ut **O**f **P**lane (OOP))
Estimated local anaesthetic volume	Suggested volumes of local anaesthetics

Abbreviations

°	degree
€	euro
λ	wavelength
ADC	analogue-to-digital converter
ASRA	American Societies of Regional Anaesthesia and Pain Medicine
BMI	body mass index
c	propagation speed
CI	confidence interval
cm	centimetre
CPR	cardiopulmonary resuscitation
CW	continuous-wave
2D	two-dimensional
3D	three-dimensional
dB	decibel
ED	effective dose
e.g	for example (*exampli gratia*)
ESRA	European Societies of Regional Anaesthesia and Pain Therapy
f	frequency
GPS	global positioning system
h	hour
Hz	Hertz
i.e.	that is (*id est*)
IIM	internal intercostal membrane
IP	in-plane
kg	kilogram
kHz	kilohertz
LA	local anaesthetic
LOR	loss-of-resistance
m	metre
mA	milliampere
mg	milligram
MHz	megahertz
min	minute
mL	millilitre
mm	millimetre
m/s	metre per second
μs	microsecond
mV	millivolt
OOP	out-of-plane
OR	operating room
PRF	pulse repetition frequency
PRI	pulse repetition interval
PW	pulsed-wave
ROI	region of interest
s	second
TAP	transversus abdominis plane
TGC	time-gain compensation
THI	tissue harmonic imaging
TPVS	thoracic paravertebral space
USA	United States of America
USB	universal serial bus
V	volts

Chapter 1

Basic principles of ultrasonography

In order to achieve ultrasound images of sufficiently high quality for regional anaesthetic peripheral nerve block techniques, some initial considerations about basic principles of ultrasonography are mandatory. The following sections outline essential knowledge required about this important topic.

1.1 Nature of sound waves

Sound is the propagation of pressure waves or an alternating series of localized regions of compression (increased pressure) and rarefaction (decreased pressure) in a material medium (e.g. air or water). Sound waves are *longitudinal*, meaning that the disturbance (alternating compression and rarefaction) occurs along the direction of propagation.

If the propagating disturbance is sinusoidal, the sound wave is composed of a single frequency (f), the rate at which successive compressions or rarefactions occur at a particular location. The units of frequency are the number of compressions (or rarefactions) per second (s) or Hertz (Hz). Besides the propagation direction and frequency, sound waves are characterized by their propagation speed (c) and wavelength (λ). The wavelength of a sound wave is defined as the geometric distance (e.g. in metres (m)) between successive regions of compression or rarefaction. The propagation speed depends on the mechanical properties of the medium (e.g. density) and varies considerably across different materials (see Table 2). The relationship between the propagation speed, frequency, and wavelength is governed by the following equation:

$$c = \lambda f$$

Audible sound (i.e. sound to which the human ear is sensitive) corresponds to frequencies ranging from 20 to 20,000Hz. Frequencies above this range are dubbed 'ultrasound', and medical imaging applications typically employ ultrasound frequencies in the range of 1 to 20MHz (i.e. up to 1,000 times higher than the human ear can hear). Since the speed of sound in human tissue is approximately 1,540m/s, the wavelengths are typically a few tenths of a millimetre.

Table 2 Speed of sound in different media

Medium	Speed of sound (m/s)
Air	333
Water	1,480
Blood	1,566
Muscle	1,542–1,626
Liver	1,566
Bone	2,070–5,350

When sound waves impinge on an interface (a location where the speed of sound changes) or propagate though a dissipative medium, some of the wave energy is scattered or deflected in multiple directions. The original wave is thus attenuated (i.e. loses energy) and the scattered energy ('echoes') carries information about the structure of the medium (e.g. that it contains an interface). It is this information that is ultimately used to create ultrasound images.

1.2 Piezoelectric effect

Some materials, notably crystals and certain ceramics, can generate an electrical voltage in response to an applied mechanical stress; these materials also exhibit the converse effect whereby their shape mechanically deforms when subjected to an electrical field. These phenomena are commonly referred to as the *piezoelectric effect* and this type of material is called piezoelectric material (Figure 1.1).

An ultrasonic transducer made out of piezoelectric materials serves as both a sound transmitter and receiver for medical imaging applications. During the sound transmission process, an electric voltage signal (typically up to 100 volts (V) or more) is converted into sound energy (i.e. stress/pressure waves) by the transducer. The generated sound wave then propagates into and interacts with the tissue under examination, and is reflected or scattered by the tissue structure. The energy received from the resulting echoes carries information about the structure, and is converted back into an electrical signal by the transducer for further processing to create ultrasound images that convey the information.

1.3 Pulse-echo instrumentation

Ultrasound images are created by transmitting and receiving a sequence of short pulses along beams spanning an anatomical region of interest (ROI).

A typical pulse (relative amplitude vs time) is shown in Figure 1.2. For each pulse, the tissue information at a particular depth is derived from the strength

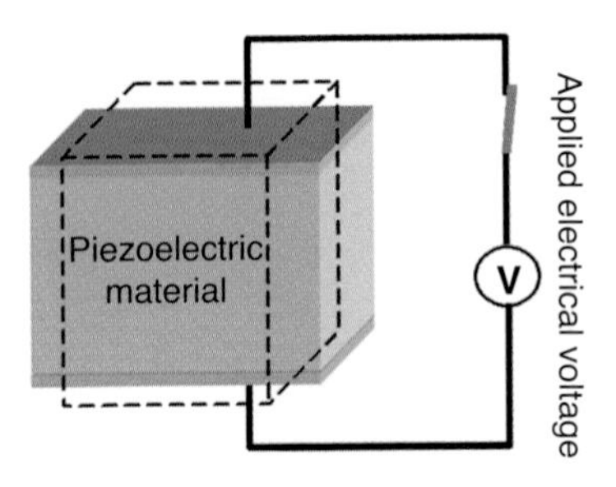

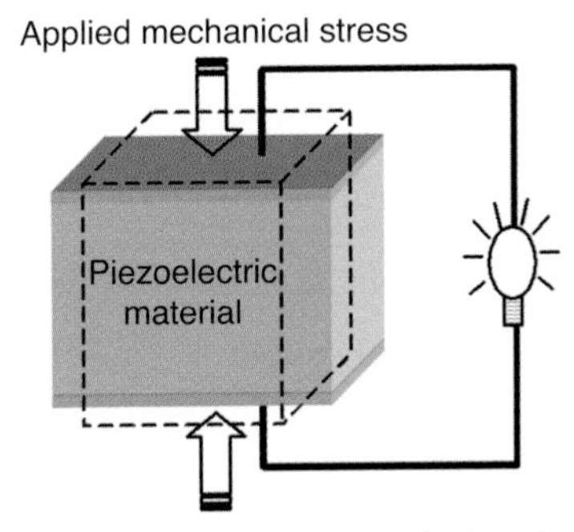

Fig. 1.1 Piezoelectric effect.

of the received echoes as a function of time. The echoes returned from each transmitted pulse are initially registered as a small voltage (100mV or less) on the individual piezoelectric elements, which is then amplified and filtered to reduce noise before being digitized with high-precision analogue-to-digital converters (ADCs). The digital signals from the individual elements are then combined to form a focused *receive beam*. Digital filtering and additional signal processing are employed to calculate the signal power as a function of time and to produce the image greyscale values along the beam direction.

The depth of an echo signal received at a particular time after transmission of the ultrasound pulse can be calculated by assuming an average speed of sound in the body, typically 1,540m/s. For example, a signal received 40μs after the pulse transmission corresponds to a depth of 3.08cm (20μs travel time each way x 1,540m/s = 0.0308m = 3.08cm). In practice, an ultrasound probe with a frequency of 13MHz allows a penetration depth of 3–4cm. A 17MHz probe with such a penetration depth would be incorrectly labelled (the manufacturer indicates in those cases the receiving, and not the transmitting, frequency).

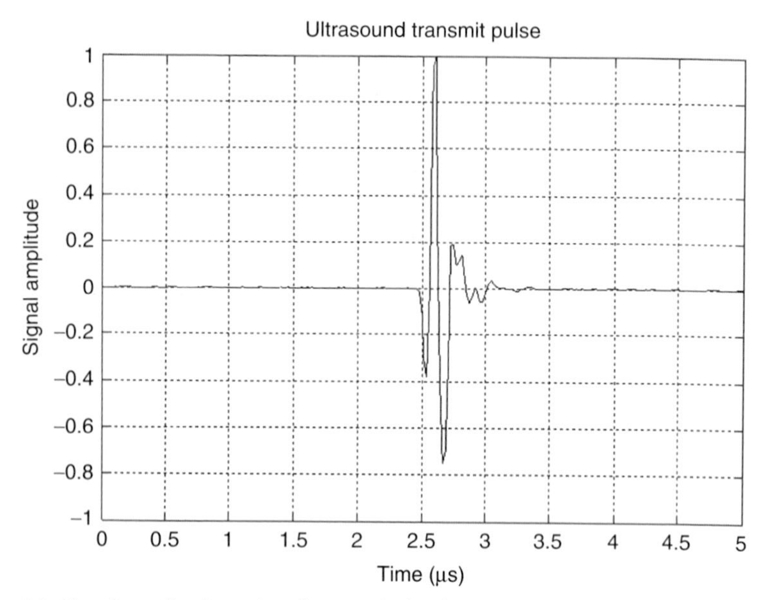

Fig. 1.2 Signal amplitude vs time for a typical pulse used in ultrasound imaging.

The image formation process is depicted in Figure 1.3, where the signal from a beam along the dotted line in the image on the right is plotted as a function of time (left), along with the detected power vs the corresponding depth (centre). The detected power values are then mapped to image greyscale values vs depth. This is repeated for each beam across the ROI to complete the image for a single frame.

1.4 **Resolution and electronic focusing**

The utility of medical images is largely determined by how well various features may be identified and distinguished from each other and from the background. The *resolution* of an image quantifies the minimum distance required between two features for them to be discriminated and may be expressed in terms of several individual components, including axial, lateral, contrast, and temporal resolution.

Axial resolution (i.e. along the line of acoustic propagation) is primarily determined by the length of the transmitted pulse. Figure 1.4 illustrates what happens when the distance between two features approaches the pulse length: they appear to fuse into a single, thicker feature, and are therefore not resolved. Higher-frequency transducers generally provide better axial resolution because higher frequencies imply shorter wavelengths which allow shorter

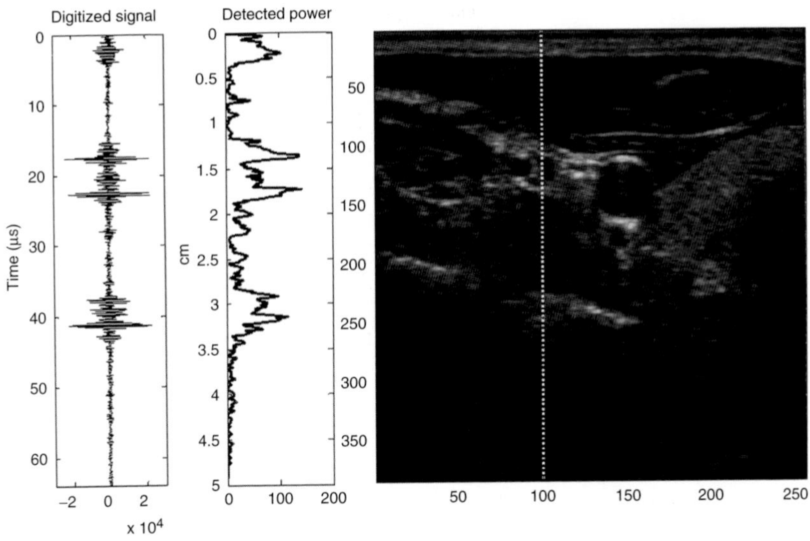

Fig. 1.3 Image formation process. The signal from a beam along the dotted line in the image (right) is plotted as a function of time (left), along with the detected power vs the corresponding depth (centre), which is then mapped to grey scale value in the image. The complete image for a single frame is formed by repeating this process for each beam across the ROI.

pulse lengths. Longer pulses are sometimes employed to increase penetration or sensitivity (since they have more energy) at the cost of degraded axial resolution.

Lateral resolution (i.e. perpendicular to the direction of acoustic propagation) is primarily determined by the focusing power of the transmitted and received beams. Ultrasound transducers for traditional 2D imaging consist of an array of individual elements arranged along a common plane, wherein each element transmits and receives ultrasound energy over a wide range of angles. A lens affixed to the front of the piezoelectric material focuses the ultrasound energy to (and from) a narrow range of elevation (the elevation direction is perpendicular to the imaging plane). To construct an image, the data from the elements are combined to form beams that focus the energy to a very narrow range of angles in the imaging plane. This is accomplished for both transmit and receive beams by summing delayed versions of the signals from the various elements. As illustrated in Figure 1.5, the delays are designed so that the propagation times from all elements to the focal point are identical. Transmit beams are focused at one of a few (typically 1–4) focal depths in the image; each requires a separate pulse, so frame rate is sacrificed for the improved

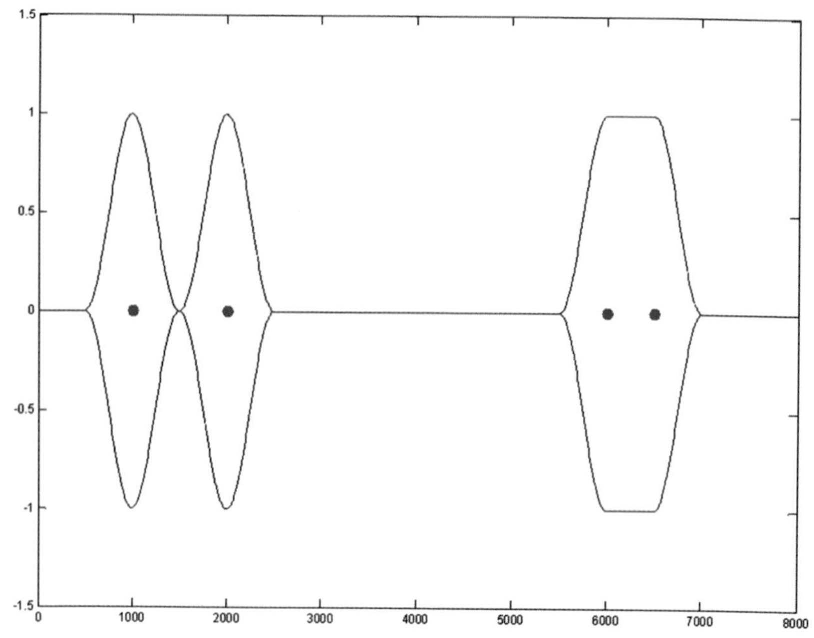

Fig. 1.4 Envelope of received signal from axially-resolved (left) and unresolved (right) pins.

resolution provided by additional transmit focal zones. Upon reception, the delays are adjusted 'dynamically' so that every point along the beam is a receive focal point.

Contrast resolution is the ability to distinguish regions of different acoustic reflectivity, as observed in the intensity or greyscale presentation of the image. The ability to detect small features or to identify small details in an image is primarily determined by a combination of spatial and contrast resolution.

Temporal resolution is the ability to track motion from frame to frame and is primarily determined by the frame rate.

1.5 **Time-gain compensation**

As an ultrasound pulse propagates through tissue, some of its energy is scattered and absorbed. This reduces the energy of the pulse as well as that of the echoes used to form an image. Because this attenuation causes the amplitude of the received signal to decrease with increasing depth, an amplifier with time-dependent gain is typically used to compensate. This ensures that the analogue signal amplitude remains in a reasonable range and prevents a

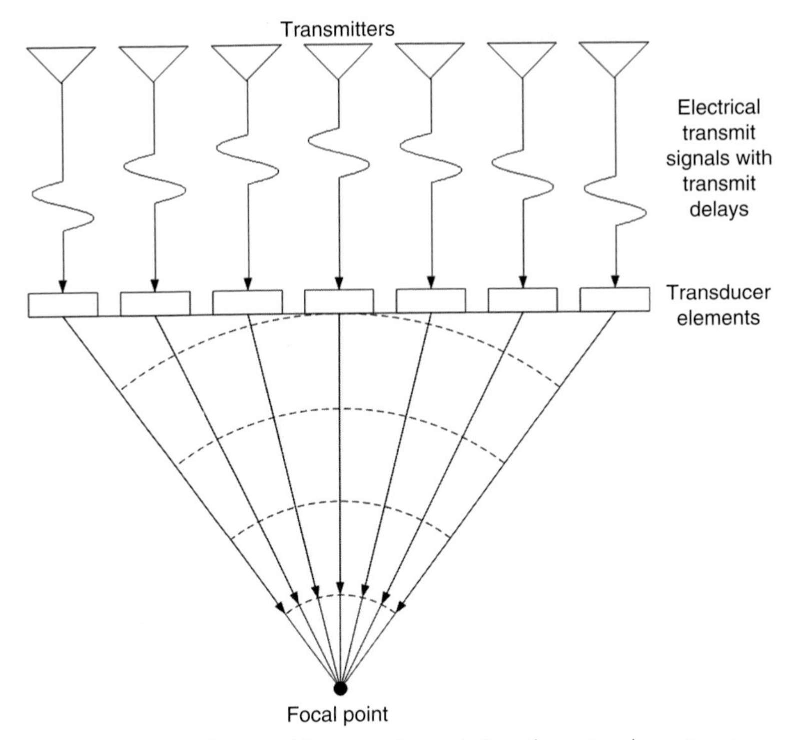

Fig. 1.5 To focus an ultrasound beam on transmission, the outer elements are pulsed before the inner elements so that the sound pulses from each element arrive at the focal point at the same time. When receiving, the signals from the outer elements are delayed relative to the inner elements before summing to compensate for the longer ultrasound path length.

reduction in image intensity with depth. As illustrated in Table 3, attenuation varies considerably across different tissue types and is usually quantified in terms of decibels (dB) per cm per MHz (where the frequency refers to the average frequency of the pulse). Typically, an average attenuation of approximately 0.5dB/cm/MHz is assumed to establish the default time-gain compensation (TGC), which can be as much as 60dB (1000-fold amplification) or more. Because attenuation varies so much with anatomy and so on, user-adjustable controls are common. For example, slide controls may allow the user to modify the gain at different depths to balance the intensity-depth profile of the image. Alternatively, some systems provide an automatic gain feature that analyzes the image data and automatically adjusts the gain as a function of depth, as shown in Figure 1.6.

Table 3 Ultrasound attenuation in various tissues

Tissues	Attenuation (dB/cm/MHz)
Water	0.0002
Blood	0.18
Soft tissues	0.3–0.8
Brain	0.3–0.5
Liver	0.4–0.7
Fat	0.5–1.8
Muscle	0.2–0.6
Tendon	0.9–1.1
Bone	13–26
Lung	40

1.6 Measuring velocity with pulsed ultrasound

The velocity of an ultrasound scatterer (e.g. a blood particle) moving along the ultrasound beam direction may be measured by correlating the reflected pulse echoes from successive transmissions ('pings'). In practice, this is accomplished by sequentially transmitting a number of beams along a fixed direction with a carefully selected, constant time interval between them. The time interval (*pulse repetition interval* (PRI) or equivalently its inverse, the *pulse repetition frequency* (PRF)), determines the velocity range that can be unambiguously estimated. For a given ultrasound frequency, the velocity range increases with increasing PRF. Ultimately, the PRF (and therefore, the maximum measurable velocity) is limited by the round trip acoustic travel time to the depth of interest because a second pulse cannot be transmitted until the first has been fully received.

Figure 1.7 illustrates how the pulse correlation technique works for two case examples: a scatterer moving away from the transducer with a relatively high velocity (Figure 1.7a, b; top panels) and a relatively low velocity (Figure 1.7a, b; bottom panels). For each, a series of received echoes is displayed (Figure 1.7a). Successive pulses are shifted in time relative to their predecessors because the object from which they are reflected is moving away from the transducer. The time shift is greater for the fast-moving scatterer because it moves further during the interval between successive pings. The right panel shows the pulse amplitude at a particular point, relative to the transmission time. These amplitude samples trace out a sinusoidal pattern with respect to the pulse index and the frequency of the sinusoid is directly proportional to the velocity of the scatterer. Ultrasound systems employ sophisticated signal processing methods to

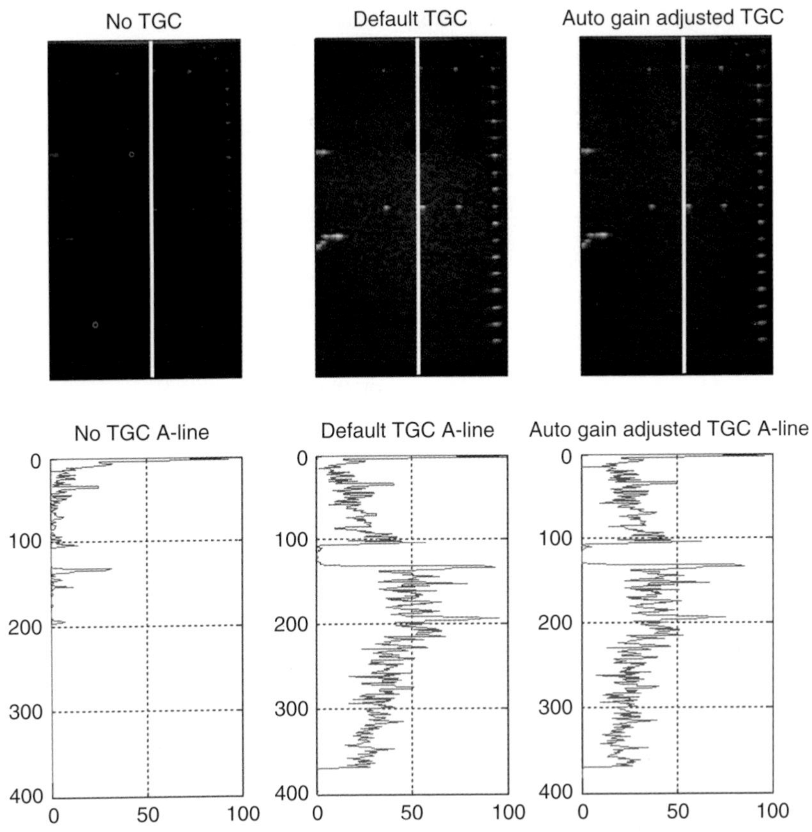

Fig. 1.6 Phantom images (top) and profiles (bottom) showing the effects of attenuation with no TGC (left), default TGC (centre), and TGC after automatic adjustment (right).

extract this information from a sequence of pulses, and use it to compute and display the spatial distribution of average velocity (*colour-flow* or *colour-velocity imaging*) or the velocity distribution of a collection of scatterers at a particular spatial location ('sample volume') as a function of time (*spectral Doppler imaging*).

1.7 **Ultrasound imaging modes**

Modern scanners present ultrasound data to doctors and sonographers in various forms. The most common form is the sonogram or *B-mode* image. An example is shown in Figure 1.8, where the 2D sector image is similar to a black and white picture of an anatomical slice.

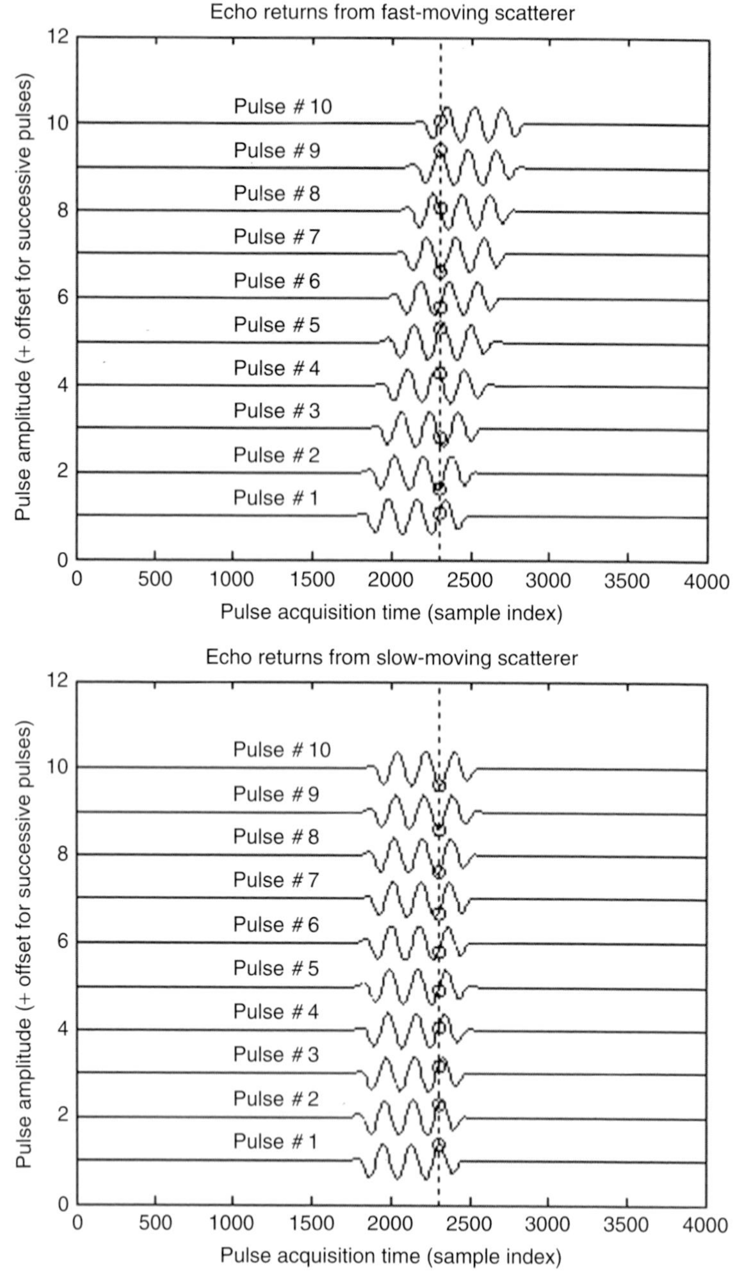

Fig. 1.7a Received echo (RF) time series reflected from a particle moving away from the transducer with relatively high velocity (top) and relatively low velocity (bottom).

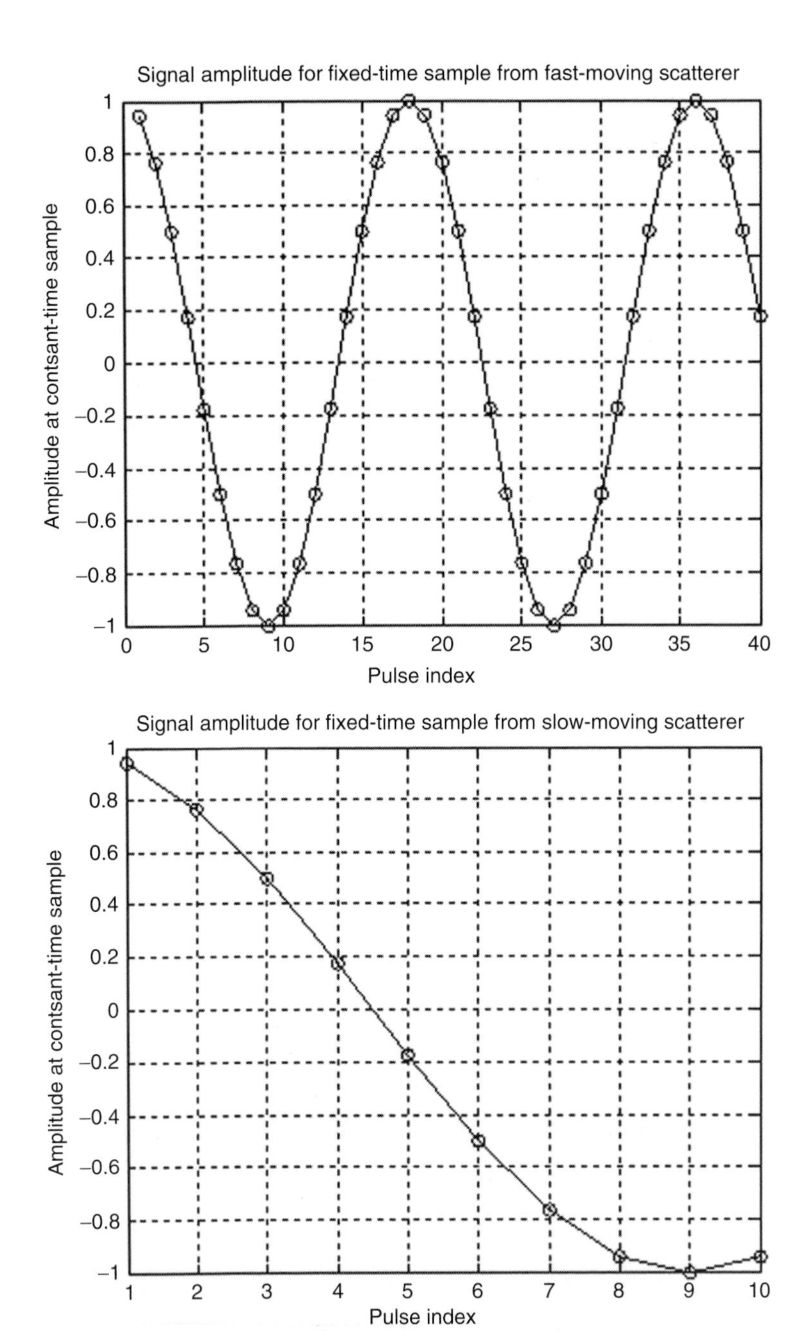

Fig. 1.7b Pulse amplitude at a fixed time relative to the transmission time for the pulses shown in Fig. 1.7a. The frequency of the resulting sinusoid is proportional to the particle velocity.

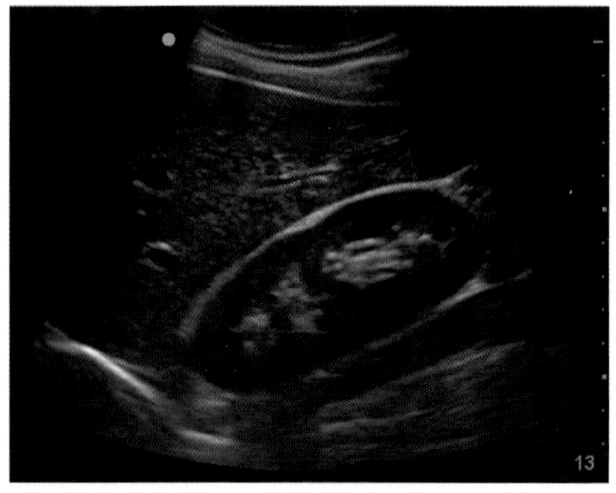

Fig. 1.8 B-mode image of the liver and kidney.

M-mode is a specialized case of B-mode imaging where one particular line (the 'm-line') is ensonified repeatedly, with the resulting greyscale information displayed as a scrolling image so that the same location is seen as it changes in time. An example is shown in Figure 1.9.

In *C-mode*, the (directional) blood velocity is estimated within an ROI and encoded as a colour image superimposed on the B-mode greyscale image, as shown in Figure 1.10. An alternative to this colour-velocity imaging is colour-flow imaging, in which the power of the blood flow signal may be displayed instead of the velocity.

An example of a *D-mode*, or spectral Doppler, image is shown in Figure 1.11. The lower portion of the figure shows a scrolling greyscale image which depicts

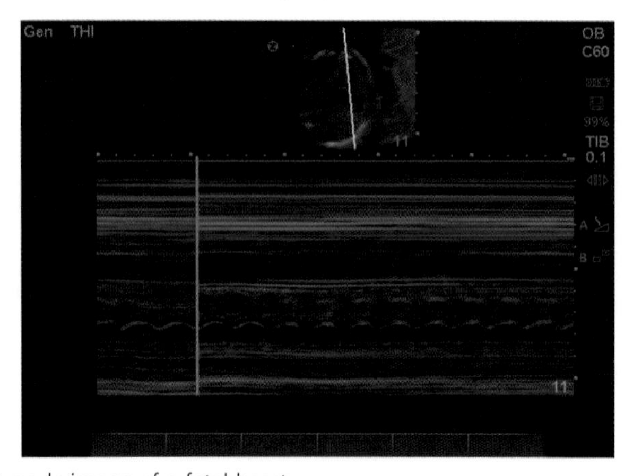

Fig. 1.9 M-mode image of a fetal heart.

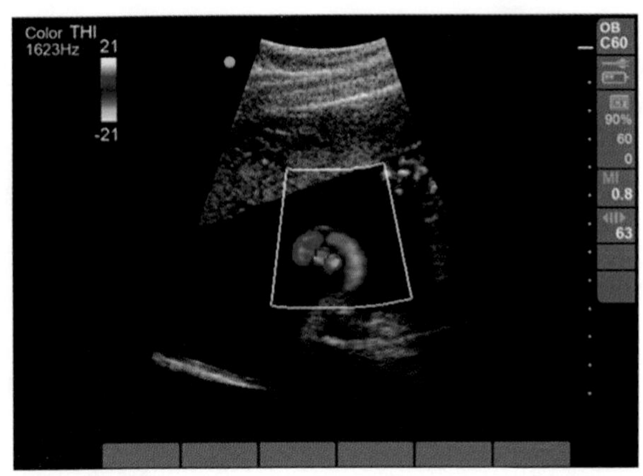

Fig. 1.10 Umbilical cord showing blood flow. Red and blue imply blood flow away from the transducer and towards the transducer, respectively.

the velocity distribution of the blood at a particular location (the *sample volume*) vs time. The vertical axis of the scrolling data represents blood velocity and the intensity (greyscale) indicates the strength of the blood flow signal. Pulsed-wave (PW) Doppler velocity ranges are limited by the depth of the sample volume.

In continuous-wave (CW) Doppler imaging, no sample volume is selected. Indeed, it is not possible to specify a time/range gate, so the velocity distribution displayed is sensitive to all depths along the selected direction. CW mode is used when the velocity range required is not accessible with PW, as it often occurs in cardiac applications. A CW Doppler image is displayed using the same format as a PW Doppler image.

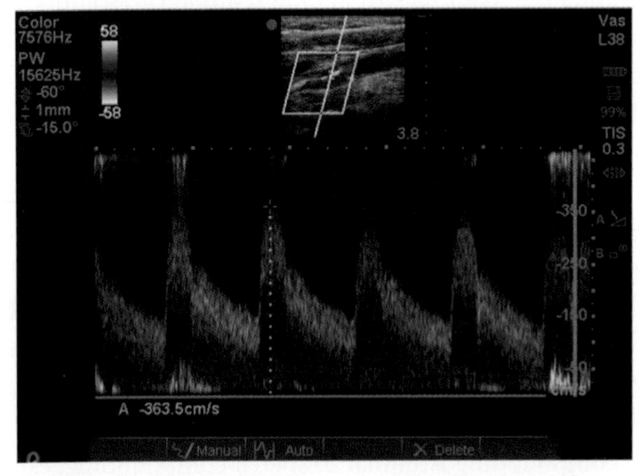

Fig. 1.11 Arterial flow in the carotid measured with spectral Doppler.

Other modalities that are increasingly common include 3D (which takes several contiguous B-mode slices and stacks them together to create a volume image), contrast imaging, and elastography. The latter entails the estimation and display of parametric images corresponding to mechanical properties of the ensonified tissue such as 'stiffness' that have been shown to correlate well with various pathology.

1.8 **Common image artefacts**

There are a number of common image artefacts that often degrade ultrasound image quality, including speckle, clutter, reverberation, and aliasing (for colour-flow and spectral Doppler). Other artefacts, such as posterior enhancement or shadowing, may also contain useful anatomical or diagnostic information. Posterior enhancement occurs when the ensonified tissue contains hypoechoic regions such as cysts or blood vessels. Hypoechoic regions reflect less ultrasound energy than the surrounding tissue. Hence, the energy remaining in the beam is significantly stronger in the region posterior to such regions and the resulting image is brighter there. Similarly, hyperechoic structures such as bones or other prominent interfaces substantially deplete the energy of the ultrasound beam and result in 'shadowing' or dark regions in the image posterior to the structures.

Speckle is a very characteristic texture commonly seen in ultrasound images. It is essentially an interference pattern superimposed on the 'true' image arising from scatterers that are too small and closely spaced to be individually resolved. Several techniques have been developed to suppress speckle and to mitigate the decreased contrast resolution it causes, including spatial compounding, frequency compounding, and image processing. The primary objective of these techniques is to increase the contrast resolution of the image while maintaining the required spatial (and temporal) resolution. All of them are commonly employed on modern, high-quality ultrasound scanners.

Spatial compounding consists of acquiring multiple image frames using ultrasound beams that are steered at different angles with respect to the surface of the transducer (without spatial compounding, all beams are typically transmitted and received perpendicular to the transducer face for 2D imaging). Because the speckle pattern varies by steering angle, the speckle from the differently steered frames is suppressed when they are registered (aligned) and combined. Typically, the number of steer directions employed varies from approximately three to nine; increasing the number of steer directions decreases speckle, but reduces the (compounded) frame rate. Figure 1.12 shows an example of the speckle suppression provided by spatial compounding.

Frequency compounding is similar to spatial compounding, except that the combined image frames are produced by using multiple (typically two) digital

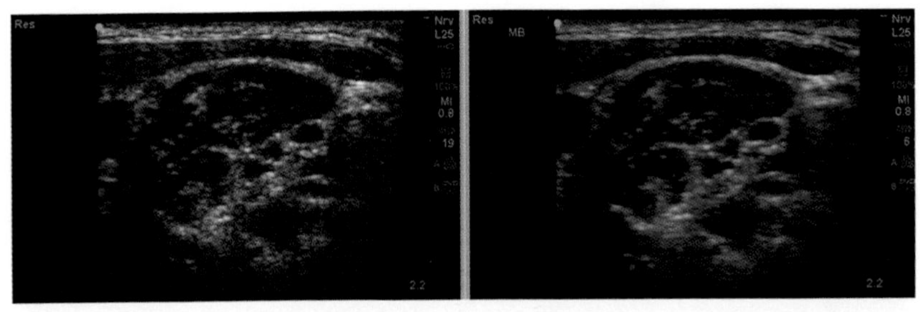

Fig. 1.12 Much of the speckle in a conventional ultrasound image (left) is suppressed in the corresponding image acquired with spatial compounding (right).

receive filters tuned to different frequencies. As with spatial compounding, the images produced from the different frequency channels contain different speckle patterns; the speckle is thus suppressed when the images are combined. Even further speckle reduction can be accomplished by combining (or substituting) spatial and frequency compounding with real-time image processing (i.e. processing applied at the acquisition rate during live scanning). Sophisticated non-linear and adaptive (i.e. image-dependent) techniques are employed on many ultrasound systems to preserve (or even enhance) detail resolution while improving contrast resolution. Figure 1.13 shows an example of an image produced with and without the application of such processing.

Although the focusing techniques described in Section 1.4 result in beams with very narrow main lobes, there may still be significant sensitivity to ultrasound energy arriving from particular directions outside of the main beam (e.g. from side or grating lobes). Echoes received from these directions will be misplaced in the image and contribute to clutter artefacts, particularly in hypoechoic regions such as vessels, amniotic fluid, cysts, and bladders. Tissue harmonic imaging (THI) and aperture apodization are frequently used to reduce these artefacts. Figure 1.14 shows how THI reduces clutter in the gall bladder.

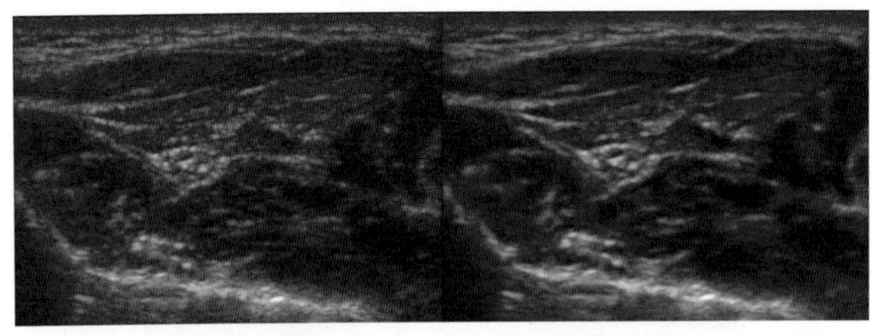

Fig. 1.13 Spatial-compounded image before (left) and after (right) speckle-reduction image processing.

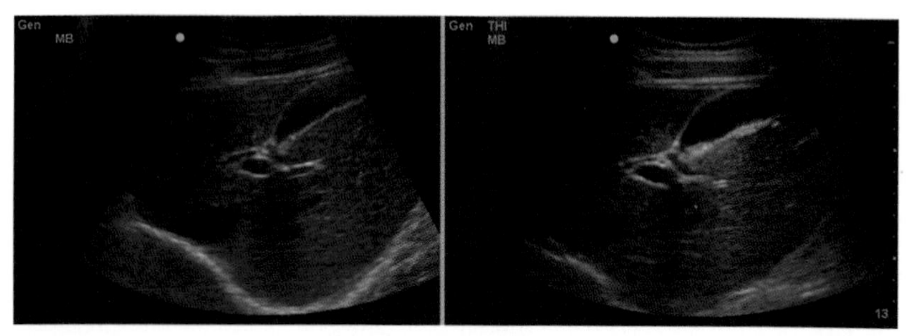

Fig. 1.14 The clutter (low-level greys) visible in the gall bladder (left) is significantly reduced in the image acquired with THI (right).

Reverberation is produced when a strong ultrasound signal is reflected back and forth between two or more interfaces with large acoustic impedance differences such as at a tissue-gas or tissue-fluid interface. A reverberation artefact typically appears as a repeated pattern of an anatomical or artificial feature (Figure 1.15).

Velocity aliasing is the most common artefact seen in colour-flow and spectral Doppler images. When the actual flow velocity is faster than the velocity a PRF can support, the aliased velocity wraps around and shows up at the opposite end of the frequency axis, as shown in Figure 1.16. A similar effect in colour-velocity images appears as artefactual reversed directional flow. Aliasing can be avoided by increasing the PRF.

1.9 Needle visualization

The ability to visualize needles is critical for guided procedures such as regional anaesthesia. For in-plane (IP) needle guidance (the needle oriented along the long axis of the transducer), most of the ultrasound energy that impinges on a needle undergoes specular reflection, as illustrated in Figure 1.17.

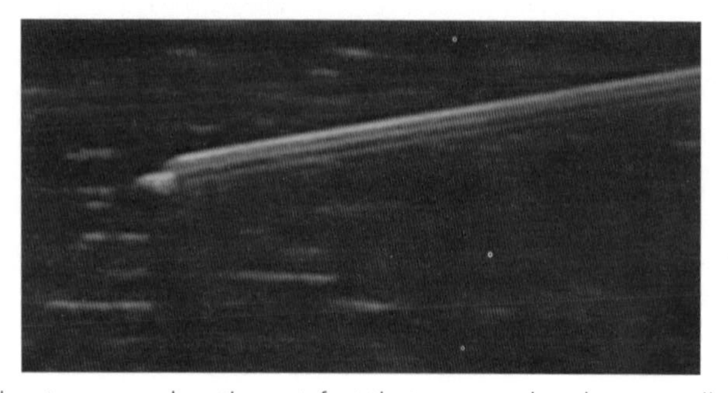

Fig. 1.15 The strong reverberation artefact that appears dorsal to a needle shaft.

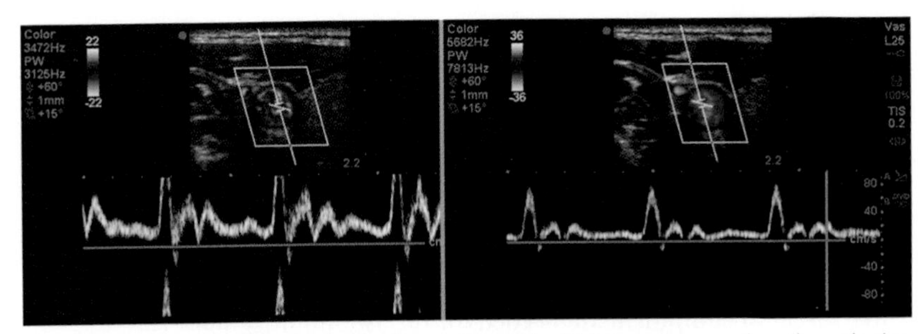

Fig. 1.16 By increasing colour velocity and Doppler PRF to proper scales, the velocity aliasing artefact (left) is diminished (right) in both imaging modes.

Since the needles are tilted with respect to the transducer surface, ultrasound beams emitted perpendicular to this surface are preferentially reflected away from the beam direction. Since there is then little needle-echo energy in the beam, the needle signal in the resulting image is weak and the needle is difficult to see. With steered beams like those used in spatial compounding, the transmitted and reflected beams (which typically coincide) are often nearly perpendicular to the needle. The reflected echoes are therefore readily detected at those steering angles and this enhanced needle signal significantly contributes to the compounded image. Needle visualization is therefore often substantially improved by spatial compounding.

Because of its importance for a variety of guided procedures, enhanced needle visualization is an active area of research and development. Many different

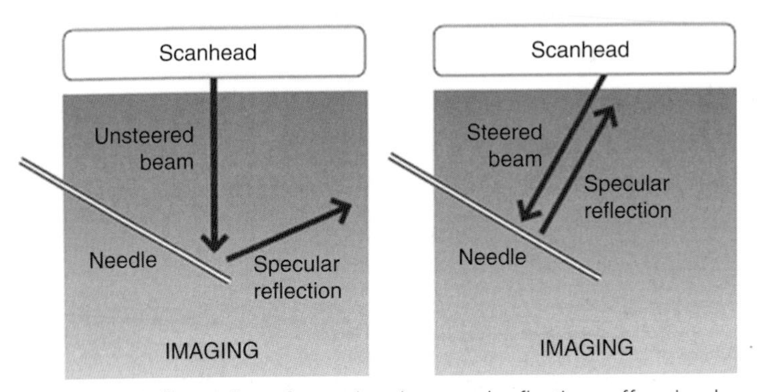

Fig. 1.17 Schematic illustration of specular ultrasound reflections off an in-plane needle from an unsteered beam (left) compared to a steered beam (right) like those used in spatial compounding. In this example, the steered beam is perpendicular to the needle, so it coincides with the direction of the specular reflection. This greatly enhances the strength of the detected signal and makes the needle easier to visualize.

approaches have been developed and commercialized to varying degrees, including those based on needles specially fabricated to enhance ultrasound reflectivity, 'smart' needle guides that sense the needle position, motion detection from ultrasound data, and automated detection by computational image processing and analysis.

1.10 Equipment needed for ultrasound imaging

Three pieces of equipment are needed for ultrasound imaging:

1) An imaging system.
2) A transducer (also known as a 'scanhead' or 'probe').
3) Transmission gel.

The system itself consists of a front-end subsystem that orchestrates the transmission signalling and reception of the reflected echoes. Transmission signalling includes pulse characteristics (e.g. centre frequency, length, and amplitude), transmit beam-forming, and the order in which beams are transmitted to compose an imaging frame. Reception includes TGC, analogue filtering, receive beam-forming, analogue-to-digital conversion, digital filtering, and various amounts of mode-specific signal processing. Additional processing is typically required to condition the data for display. System software is also required to:

1) Provide a user interface that allows the user to select imaging mode, depth, exam type, etc.
2) Configure the various system components based on these inputs.
3) Provide connectivity (e.g. internet, USB, and so on).
4) Perform various calculations based on the ultrasound data and/or additional user inputs.

Three types of transducers are used for the vast majority of 2D ultrasound imaging applications:

1) Linear arrays (Figure 1.18).
2) Curved arrays (Figure 1.19).
3) Phased arrays.

High-frequency probes provide superior spatial resolution whereas low-frequency probes offer greater penetration. Linear arrays are typically used to produce images with a finely sampled, rectangular field of view whereas curved arrays are typically used to produce a diverging 'sector-shaped' field of view that expands beyond the lateral extent of the transducer. Phased arrays often

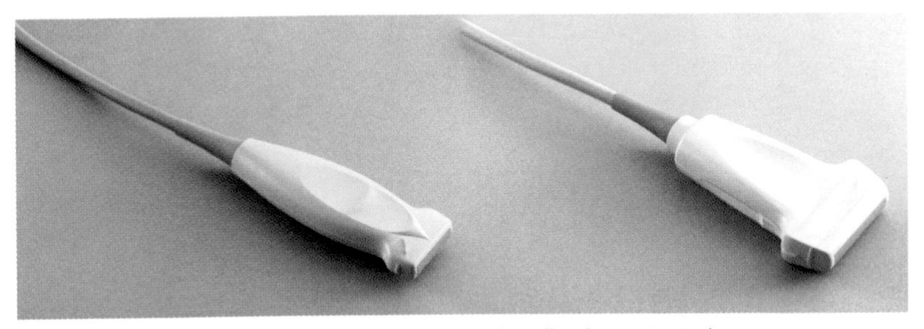

Fig. 1.18 25 and 38mm linear ultrasound probes (both 6–13MHz).

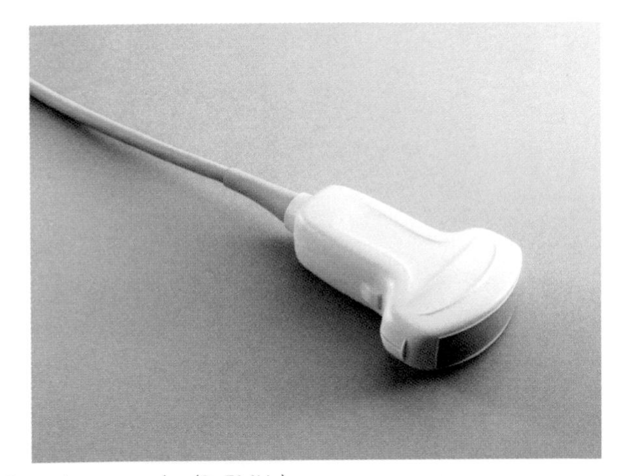

Fig. 1.19 Curved array probe (2–5MHz).

provide a linear array 'form factor' with the expanding field of view that is characteristic of curved arrays.

Transmission gel is essential for ultrasound imaging. Without it, there would inevitably be an air gap between the surface of the transducer and the patient. Because the speed of sound is so different in air, most of the ultrasound energy would be reflected from this interface and would not propagate into the patient. Gel provides a coupling medium that efficiently transmits ultrasound energy from the transducer to the patient and vice versa.

Chapter 2

The scientific background of ultrasound guidance in regional anaesthesia

An adequate scientific evaluation is necessary to translate a new technique into daily clinical practice. Starting with simple descriptions of block techniques from the mid-nineties, it became more and more obvious that ultrasound guidance in regional anaesthesia offers a lot of advantages, but is also associated with drawbacks. Today a large number of different ultrasound-guided regional techniques are described and physicians from all over the world are interested to use these techniques in their daily clinical practice. This increasing interest is associated with an enormous responsibility for clinical scientists. It is a matter of fact that not all descriptions of block techniques are clinically useful and some are obviously dangerous. While ultrasound-guided, intraneuronal injection of local anaesthetic serves as the most dangerous description, other techniques such as the posterior approach to the interscalene brachial plexus are simply not useful from a practical and anatomical point of view (see specific chapters).

Today we are able to move more and more into volunteer studies. The investigation of important questions is more effective by using volunteers as compared with a clinical study setting where patients are under serious stress due to pain and apprehension with the forthcoming surgical procedure. In addition, data acquisition is much more reliable in volunteers. Investigations regarding the volume reduction of local anaesthetics are one example of a highly sophisticated study setting which aims to increase the safety of regional blocks. Such volume reduction studies in a clinical setting are associated with ethical problems where block failures with the need for additional anaesthesia techniques are *prima vista* included in the study protocol. On the other hand, volunteers will not undergo surgery and therefore, the ultimate evidence for a successful block—the surgical procedure—is not investigated in those study settings. Therefore, we face the dilemma that maximal reliable clinical data are required without the knowledge regarding an 'optimal' study design.

Pharmacological studies in the field of regional anaesthesia are one solution to increase the understanding about regional anaesthetic block mechanism and to answer particular questions. A recent study by Weintraud et al. investigates the serum levels of local anaesthetic during ultrasound compared with the landmark-based ilioinguinal-iliohypogastric nerve blockade in children. The serum levels were significantly lower when a landmark-based technique is used for this abdominal wall block. This makes sense since in most of these cases, the local anaesthetic is administered inside muscles whereas the ultrasound-guided technique is associated with an exact administration of the local anaesthetic between muscle tissues with subsequent larger contact areas between the local anaesthetic and surrounding tissue. The results of this study support the demand of low volumes of local anaesthetics when ultrasound is used.

But scientific studies should not only answer specific questions in the field of ultrasound-guided regional anaesthesia techniques. There is a requirement to design studies to answer the ultimate question: Does ultrasound increase the safety of regional anaesthetic blocks? Considering the fact that regional anaesthesia is a safe specialty regarding severe complications, a hundred thousand cases will be required for these studies. Thus, a multicentre study design will be an essential prerequisite for the investigation of safety issues. These studies will influence the daily clinical practice in the most significant way.

Suggested further reading

Latzke, D., Marhofer, P., Zeitlinger, M., Machata, A., Neumann, F., Lackner, E., Kettner, S.C., 2010. Minimal local anaesthetic volumes for sciatic nerve block: evaluation of ED99 in volunteers. *British Journal of Anaesthesia* 104(2), pp.239–44.

Weintraud, M., Lundblad, M., Kettner, S.C., Willschke, H., Kapral, S., Lönnqvist, P.A., Koppatz, K., Turnheim, K., Bösenberg, A., Marhofer, P., 2009. Ultrasound versus landmark-based technique for ilioinguinal-iliohypogastric nerve blockade in children: the implications on plasma levels of ropivacaine. *Anesthesia & Analgesia*, 108(5), pp.1488–92.

Chapter 3

Initial considerations and potential advantages of regional anaesthesia under ultrasound guidance

3.1 History of ultrasound-guided regional anaesthesia

Undoubtedly, ultrasonography has influenced the subspecialty of regional anaesthesia during the past 15 years. Progress from the year 1884 when Carl Koller performed the first regional block for eye surgery in Vienna to the late 1970s was rather slow. The main findings during that time were based on the development of new local anaesthetic solutions and morphometric methods of nerve identification. Anatomical considerations were poor with subsequently weak success rates. The significant concerns against regional anaesthesia are perhaps dated from those times.

It is an interesting observation that 'regional anaesthesiologists' have developed their own ideas of anatomy. The considerations behind the '3-in-1' block with the assumption of a fascial sheath extending from the inguinal ligament upwards to the lumbar plexus should serve as only one example of misinterpretation of the anatomical reality. Anyway, at those times, it was difficult to confirm the spread of local anaesthetics during regional blocks. Only conventional X-ray was available to diagnose the spread of fluids. The major drawback of X-ray is the impossibility of visualizing neuronal structures and therefore, only an indirect imagination of the correlation between fluids and neuronal structures was possible.

The implementation of ultrasonography in clinical practice improved this technical problem. The first manuscript in that field was published in 1978 by La Grange et al. where a Doppler ultrasound blood flow detector was used to facilitate a supraclavicular brachial plexus blockade. Obviously, knowledge about the ultrasonographic appearance of neuronal structures was weak at that time and ultrasound technology was not suitable to visualize nerves. The first direct use of ultrasound for a regional block was published by Kapral et al. in 1994, again for a supraclavicular brachial plexus blockade.

It took another ten years of development and particular considerations to achieve an adequate level of knowledge and a parallel evolution of ultrasound technology. With an increasing popularity of ultrasound in regional anaesthesia, manufacturers of ultrasound equipment designed dedicated machines and specialized software to facilitate regional blocks under ultrasonographic guidance. This led to the development of the quality of ultrasound scans increasing with the subsequent increase in the quality of blocks. As with analogue to mobile phones and other electronic equipment, ultrasound machines became smaller and cheaper. It is still the case that ultrasound machines are expensive, but recent investigations demonstrate the cost effectiveness of ultrasound-guided regional anaesthesia in daily clinical practice.

Several positive developments facilitated the use of ultrasound for regional blocks. But it is also a matter of fact that disputable techniques have been described in the past, and it is extremely difficult for the practitioner to differentiate between useful and uncertain descriptions and techniques. Clearly, it should be allowed to discuss all facets of this important topic and only the future will show if a particular description and technique is applicable in daily clinical practice. It is also clear that every article in that field (like in any other field) reflects the opinion of their authors. Therefore, large multicentre studies are required to bring light to our knowledge about advantages and drawbacks of the use of ultrasound for regional techniques. In any case, these studies will be associated with severe and possibly irreconcilable, problematic statements. The obtainment of true and verified data from a large number of study centres should serve as only one example why such a study will be difficult to realize. 'Ultrasound enthusiasts' tend to overestimate their hand skills and success of techniques whereas sworn followers of a more 'conventional' technique tend to demonize ultrasound and neglect any usefulness of new techniques. Both apodictic and arrogant points of view are inappropriate and impedimental for a fair and meaningful comparison of techniques. Much happened during the past 16 years, but in light of the aforementioned facts, it is much more important to consider what will happen during the next 20 years.

3.2 **Possible advantages of ultrasound-guided regional anaesthesia**

Several advantages, drawbacks, and controversial opinions of ultrasound-guided, regional blocks have been described in a number of well-designed studies and confirmed in clinical practice. These are discussed herein.

3.2.1 Overall safety of ultrasound-guided blocks

The main argument against ultrasound guidance for regional techniques is the lack of large, randomized studies comparing the complications of ultrasound guidance with other techniques. As the complication rate of regional anaesthesia is nowadays very low, such studies would have to include thousands of patients. Thus, we have to accept that these large outcome studies will not be available in the near (or even far) future. We should therefore try to find an acceptable midpoint between 'evidence-based' and 'expert-based' medicine concerning the use of ultrasound-guided regional anaesthesia.

The question of whether ultrasonographic guidance increases the margin of safety for regional block techniques divides the 'regional anaesthetic world' into two parts. Those who advocate for the view that direct visualization of the anatomy involved is associated with increased safety and those with a negative attitude have comprehensible arguments. Clearly, the topic regarding safety in regional anaesthesia is controversially discussed in the literature. The incidence of complications ranges from 0.0004% (Auroy et al., 2002) to 14% (Borgeat et al., 2001). Thus, an orientation regarding the true rate of complication is difficult.

Fredrickson et al. (2009) analyzed 1,010 ultrasonographic-guided blocks and found neurological symptoms in 8.2% after ten days, 3.7% after one month, and 0.6% after six months. These percentages are similar to conventional techniques. Liu et al. (2009) compared 200 interscalene blocks performed either with ultrasound or nerve stimulator guidance and observed after one week a rate of neurological complications of 8% with ultrasound and 11% with nerve stimulation. It is important to state that perioperative neurological complications may be caused by several mechanisms (positioning, tourniquet, swelling, etc.), and therefore, an evaluation of the true rate of complications caused by regional anaesthesia is difficult. Even if the current literature does not support the safety of ultrasonographic guidance in regional anaesthesia, it seems obvious that the correct use of this technique is associated with an increased margin of safety.

3.2.2 Safe identification of neuronal structures

With today's ultrasound equipment, the identification of even the smallest neuronal structures is possible. Nevertheless, an adequate technique remains an important prerequisite with individual knowledge and hand skills of equal importance. A high level of experience with ultrasonography is the most important factor for the safe identification of neuronal structures. Every nerve has a particular appearance in ultrasonography, and the shape and echogenicity of this may vary in different anatomical regions.

3.2.3 Detection of anatomical variants and variations

One of the main reasons for block failures may be caused by anatomical variations. It is important to distinguish between anatomical variants and variations. An anatomical variant represents the normal anatomy whereas an anatomical variation represents atypical (and rare) relationships between anatomical structures. The division of the sciatic nerve in the tibial and peroneal nerves is highly variable and therefore, it is an anatomical variant. The nerve roots of the brachial plexus inside the anterior scalene muscle are rather rare findings and therefore, they are anatomical variations.

Ultrasound is the only bedside method where anatomical variants and variations may be detected. The relevant anatomical variations for each topographic region are described throughout this book.

3.2.4 Identification of adjacent anatomical structures

Of particular importance for establishing safe and effective nerve blocks is the identification of any relevant adjacent anatomical structures such as vessels, bones, tendons, muscles, pleura, or lymph nodes. Puncture of the pleura during supraclavicular brachial plexus blockade with subsequent pneumothorax is a severe complication and can be safely avoided during direct visualization. The ability to identify these adjacent anatomical structures via ultrasound is *the* prerequisite to avoid inadvertent needle positions and subsequent complications.

3.2.5 Exact administration of local anaesthetic and observation of the spread of local anaesthetic

It is often forgotten that it is the local anaesthetic solution which blocks the nerve and that the distribution of local anaesthetic cannot be reliably predicted with indirect needle guidance techniques. Indeed, direct observation of the spread of local anaesthetic is one of the main advantages of ultrasonography. In cases of maldistribution of the local anaesthetic, needle replacement is always possible in order to achieve an adequate spread.

A recent publication by Weintraud et al. (2008) describes the performance of ultrasound-controlled pure landmark-orientated ilioinguinal-iliohypogastric nerve blocks in children. The authors of this investigator-blinded study performed nerve blocks in children via conventional 'fascial click' methods and observed the spread of local anaesthetic by ultrasound. In only 14% of the cases, the local anaesthetic was administered correctly between the internal oblique and transverse abdominal muscles. This study is an impressive example of the difficulties associated with landmark-based techniques.

The unpredictable spread of local anaesthetic during peripheral nerve blockade favours the *multi-injection technique* which is promoted throughout this book. The multi-injection technique should be used even for single nerve blocks. Moreover, complex regional anaesthetic techniques (e.g. interscalene or supraclavicular brachial plexus blockade) are only manageable with low volumes of local anaesthetic when multi-injections are used.

3.2.6 Observation of the needle

In addition to ensuring an adequate spread of local anaesthetic, direct observation of the needle is an important factor to avoid complications. Whether the entire needle can be visualized in its entirety or only at the tip depends on the block technique being used (IP vs OOP). Both techniques have their specific indications with associated advantages and problems (see Chapter 8). Although it is frequently stated in this book that it is the local anaesthetic and not the tip of the needle that provides a successful nerve block, direct visualization of the tip of the needle is mandatory for a successful block and the safe avoidance of complications (e.g. nerve puncture or damage of adjacent anatomical structures). These requirements are independent whether an IP or OOP technique is used.

3.2.7 Faster onset times and longer duration of blocks

Because of the close administration of local anaesthetic to nerve structures, the onset times of ultrasound-guided blocks are significantly shorter compared with conventional techniques. It has also been shown that the duration of blocks is significantly longer following ultrasound-guided techniques. These improvements in block characteristics are based on the exact administration of local anaesthetic and are, to a certain extent, independent of the volume of local anaesthetic that is used.

3.2.8 Painless performance of blocks

Ideally, regional anaesthesia is performed in a painless manner. With the sole exception of ultrasound guidance, all current techniques are based on the physical interaction with nerves (e.g. paraesthesia techniques, nerve stimulation) and are therefore associated with uncomfortable sensations. Furthermore, muscle response during nerve stimulation is a painful procedure in cases of traumas (e.g. luxation of joints, fractures). In addition, the smaller volumes of local anaesthetic required for ultrasound-guided techniques compared with conventional methods, along with the subsequent reduction in pressure forces, may provide superior comfort to patients during blockade.

Pain during regional blocks can also be reduced with the use of sharp needle tips (e.g. Facette tips) whereas blunt needles require force when the needle is advanced and may cause more tissue trauma. Appropriate sizes of needles are also useful to realize painless block procedures. Therefore, 22-G Facette tip needles are the most appropriate equipment for peripheral nerve blocks in adults and older children. Smaller needles (e.g. 24-G) are useful for blocks in children under 3 years old.

3.2.9 Reduced volumes of local anaesthetics

In addition to its pain-sparing benefits, reducing the volume of local anaesthetic used in nerve blockade also increases the safety of the procedure. Several studies have shown that blocks using 20 to 30% of previously recommended local anaesthetic volumes are possible under direct visualization of the nerve structures. It seems that large volumes have been used in the past to compensate for inaccurate guidance techniques. On reviewing the literature, one can still find recommendations to administer 60mL of local anaesthetic for interscalene or axillary brachial plexus blocks. As a consequence, side effects such as co-blockade of the phrenic nerve may occur during interscalene blockade. In addition, low (or adequate) administration of local anaesthetics reduces the risk of systemic toxicity; patients with impaired cardiovascular function may benefit from low plasma levels of local anaesthetics. This is also true for children in whom low levels of binding proteins can cause increased toxicity of local anaesthetics. Table 4 illustrates a list of publications on reduced volumes of local anaesthetics for various regional anaesthetic techniques.

3.2.10 Low complication rates and high success rates with reduced conversions to alternative anaesthetic methods

Given these potential advantages, ultrasound-guided regional anaesthesia should result in low rates of complications and high success rates. However, as mentioned earlier, it is extremely difficult to provide adequately rigorous, scientific evidence for the observed reduction of complication rates with ultrasound-guided methods in comparison with conventional techniques. Our knowledge about nerve physiology is still not sufficient to understand all the mechanisms of nerve damage and potential dangers of electro-stimulation or direct nerve puncture. Nevertheless, it seems an appropriate concept to avoid needle-nerve contact in order to prevent nerve damage. In any case, direct visualization of all anatomical structures involved in the blockade increases the safety of regional

Table 4 List of publications on volume reduction of local anaesthetic

Publication	Nerve structure	Minimum effective volume	Statistical method	Additional description
Willschke et al. (*Anesthesia & Analgesia*, 2006)	Ilioinguinal-iliohypogastric nerves	0.075mL/kg	Clinical setting, modified step-up/step-down approach	Children
Casati et al. (*British Journal of Anaesthesia*, 2007)	Femoral nerve	ED_{50} 22mL (95% CI, 13–36mL)	Clinical setting, up-and-down staircase method	Relatively large volume despite the use of ultrasound
Riazi et al. (*British Journal of Anaesthesia*, 2008)	Interscalene brachial plexus block	5mL	Clinical setting, comparative study design (5 vs 20mL)	5mL equi-effective with 20mL
Eichenberger et al. (*Regional Anesthesia and Pain Medicine*, 2009)	Ulnar nerve	ED_{95} 0.11mL/mm^2 nerve area	Experimental setting, up-and-down procedure according to the Dixon average method	Evaluation of the minimum effective volume of local anaesthetic based on the cross-sectional nerve area
O´Donnell et al. (*Anesthesiology*, 2009)	Brachial plexus (axillary approach)	1mL/nerve	Clinical setting, step-up / step-down study model	
Duggan et al. (*Regional Anesthesia and Pain Medicine*, 2009)	Supraclavicular plexus	ED_{50} 23mL, ED_{95} 42mL	Clinical setting, up-and-down procedure according to the Dixon average method	No difference to conventional methods of nerve identification
Latzke et al. (*British Journal of Anaesthesia*, 2010)	Sciatic nerve at the mid-femoral level	ED_{99} 0.10mL/mm^2 cross-sectional nerve area	Experimental setting, up-and-down procedure ccording to the Dixon average method	Evaluation of the minimum effective volume of local anaesthetic based on the cross-sectional nerve area
Marhofer et al. (*Anaesthesia*, 2010)	Brachial plexus (axillary approach)	0.11mL vs 0.4mL/mm^2 nerve area	Volunteer study, prospective, double-blinded, crossover	Longer sensory onset time in low-volume group, no statistically significant differences in duration and over success of blocks

ED: effective dose; CI: confidence interval

techniques and avoids damage to these structures during puncture. Despite a lack of adequate clinical trials, this concept for avoiding complications appears convincing.

From literature review, an overall success rate of 80% for peripheral regional techniques with conventional guidance techniques is described. This implies a large number of block failures and subsequently high conversion rates to alternative methods. Conversion to general anaesthesia is associated with patient discomfort and an increased incidence of complications. In addition, the necessity of a second anaesthesia method is uneconomical.

3.2.11 Economical aspects of ultrasound-guided blocks

There is the widespread opinion that ultrasound-guided regional techniques are extremely expensive. Clearly, ultrasound equipment is associated with significant costs, but manufacturers have started to downsize ultrasound equipment, thus resulting in cost reductions. Like other electronic equipment (mobile phones, laptop computers, GPS navigations, etc.), ultrasound equipment is also affordable nowadays. Ten years ago, it was difficult to get an adequate ultrasound machine for less than €80,000. Today, excellent equipment is available for between €20,000 and €30,000. But it is short-sighted to consider only the direct costs of ultrasound equipment in the context of the entire area of ultrasound and regional anaesthesia. A recent publication by Gonano et al. (2009) investigates the economical aspects of ultrasound-guided interscalene blocks for arthroscopic shoulder surgery. The authors of that study observed a reduction of more than €170 per case on considering direct cost effects (drugs, disposables, etc.) and workflow-related costs. The most important prerequisites to realize this cost-effective method are sufficient block success and an optimal anaesthesia-related workflow. It is important to highlight that a cost of €15/min has to be calculated for every minute in the operation room and therefore, faster anaesthesia induction and emerging times are *the* significant factors for cost reduction. Under adequate conditions, more than €100,000/year per operation room can be saved with an effective performance of ultrasound-guided regional blocks.

Suggested further reading

Auroy, Y., Benhamou, D., Bargues, L., Ecoffey, C., Falissard, B., Mercier, F.J., Bouaziz, H., Samii, K., 2002. Major complications of regional anaesthesia in France: The SOS Regional Anaesthesia Hotline Service. *Anesthesiology*, 97(5), pp.1274–80.

Borgeat, A., Ekatodramis, G., Kalberer, F., Benz, C., 2001. Acute and non-acute complications associated with interscalene block and shoulder surgery: a prospective study. *Anesthesiology*, 95(4), pp.875–80.

Eichenberger, U., Stöckli, S., Marhofer, P., Huber, G., Willimann, P., Kettner, S.C., Pleiner, J., Curatolo, M., Kapral, S., 2009. Minimal local anesthetic volume for peripheral nerve block: a new ultrasound-guided, nerve dimension-based method. *Regional Anesthesia and Pain Medicine*, 34(3), pp.242–6.

Fredrickson, M.J., Kilfoyle, D.H., 2009. Neurologicalal complication analysis of 1000 ultrasound-guided peripheral nerve blocks for elective orthopaedic surgery: a prospective study. *Anaesthesia*, 64(8), pp.836–44.

Gonano, C., Kettner, S.C., Ernstbrunner, M., Schebesta, K., Chiari, A., Marhofer, P., 2009. Comparison of economical aspects of interscalene brachial plexus blockade and general anaesthesia for arthroscopic shoulder surgery. *British Journal of Anaesthesia*, 103(3), pp.428–33.

Kapral, S., Krafft, P., Eibenberger, K., Fitzgerald, R., Gosch, M., Weinstabl, C., 1994. Ultrasound-guided supraclavicular approach for regional anaesthesia of the brachial plexus. *Anesthesia & Analgesia*, 78(3), pp.507–13.

La Grange, P., Foster, P.A., Pretorius, L.K., 1978. Application of the Doppler ultrasound bloodflow detector in supraclavicular brachial plexus block. *British Journal of Anaesthesia*, 50(9), pp.965–7.

Latzke, D., Marhofer, P., Zeitlinger, M., Machata, A., Neumann, F., Lackner, E., Kettner, S.C., 2010. Minimal local anaesthetic volumes for sciatic nerve block: evaluation of ED99 in volunteers. *British Journal of Anaesthesia*, 104(2), pp.239–44.

Liu, S.S., Zayas, V.M., Gordon, M.A., Beathe, J.C., Maalouf, D.B., Paroli, L., Liguori, G.A., Ortiz, J., Buschiazzo, V., Ngeow, J., Shetty, T., Ya Deau, J.T., 2009. A prospective, randomized, controlled trial comparing ultrasound versus nerve stimulator guidance for interscalene block for ambulatory shoulder surgery for post-operative neurological symptoms. *Anesthesia & Analgesia*, 109(1), pp.265–71.

Marhofer, P., Eichenberger, U., Stöckli, S., Huber, G., Kapral, S., Curatolo, M., Kettner, S., 2010. Ultrasonographic-guided axillary plexus blocks with low volumes of local anaesthetics: a crossover volunteer study. *Anaesthesia*, 65(3), pp.266–71.

Weintraud, M., Marhofer, P., Bosenberg, A., Kapral, S., Willschke, H., Felfernig, M., Kettner, S., 2008. Ilioinguinal/iliohypogastric blocks in children: where do we administer the local anaesthetic without direct visualization? *Anesthesia & Analgesia*, 106(1), pp.89–93.

Chapter 4

Technique limitations and suggestions for a training concept

Every serious analysis of a new method should also consider its potential limitations. For ultrasound-guided regional anaesthesia, these can be divided into technical and non-technical limitations.

4.1 Technical limitations

Physical law dictates that the deeper the anatomical structures, the lower the ultrasound frequencies needed to visualize them. Therefore, direct nerve visualization for deep blocks, such as psoas compartment blockade, is not always possible. Nevertheless, the identification of adjacent structures (e.g. the lower pole of the kidney during psoas compartment blockade) increases the margin of safety for deep blocks.

Not all regional techniques are meaningful under ultrasound guidance. A questionable regional technique for ultrasound guidance is epidural anaesthesia in adults. Since most of the neuraxial structures are surrounded and protected by bones, the ultrasound visualization of the epidural space is limited and in some cases, almost impossible. Despite extensive scientific and practical efforts of experienced users, ultrasound guidance for the placement of epidural catheters has not found its way into daily clinical practice. Whereas all neuraxial structures in children are clearly visible (Figure 4.1), albeit in an age- and weight-dependent manner, ultrasonography of neuraxial structures in adults is limited (Figure 4.2).

4.2 Non-technical limitations

In addition to these technical limitations of ultrasound-guided regional anaesthesia, one of the main challenges of increasing its usage in clinical practice is that anaesthesiologists have to change their mind. It is difficult to convince those who have worked for several years with alternative methods of nerve identification during regional blocks. Indeed, it is easy to find arguments

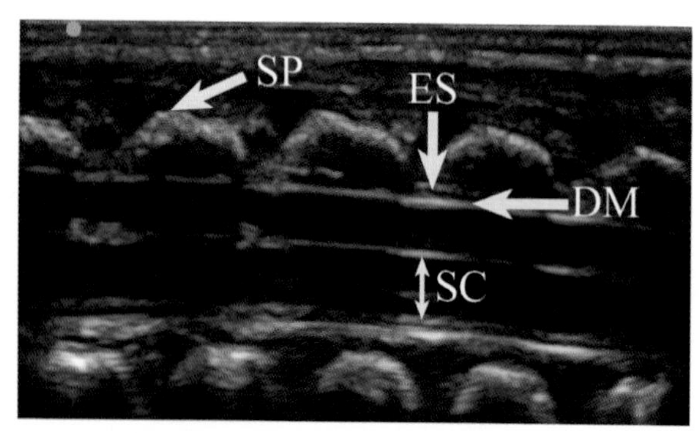

Fig. 4.1 Ultrasonographic appearance of the neuraxial structures in a 3kg baby. SC: spinal cord; DM: dura mater; ES: epidural space; SP: spinous process; left side=cranial.

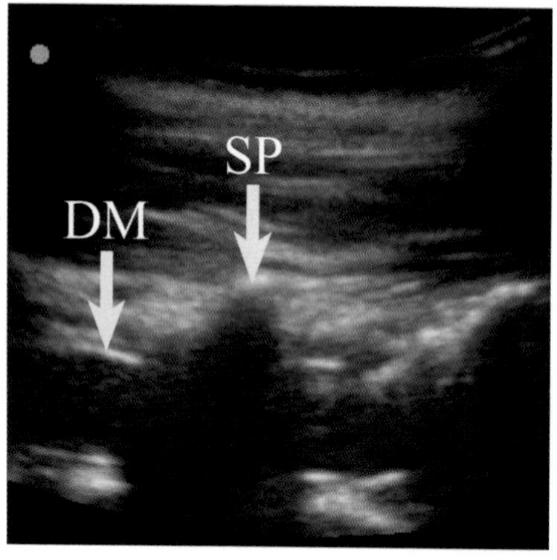

Fig. 4.2 Ultrasonographic appearance of neuraxial structures in a 30 year old adult. SP: spinous process; DM=dura mater; left side=cranial.

against new techniques, and several years of intensive, scientific, and practical evaluation are usually needed to introduce a new technique in widespread clinical practice.

4.3 Suggestions for a training concept in ultrasound-guided regional anaesthesia

A prerequisite for the adequate use of a new technique is intensive education and training. In recent years, several useful workshops have been established all over the world, both as part of anaesthesia congresses and as independent, highly specialized workshops (e.g. www.sono-nerve.com, www.nysora.com). However, the optimal method to introduce ultrasound-guided regional blockade into daily clinical practice remains under discussion. It is rather difficult to provide close supervision by experienced users for the high number of potential and interested anaesthesiologists and institutions. Therefore, optimal learning tools are prerequisites and an absolute necessity for novices and those with limited experience. Useful learning tools should include DVDs that demonstrate practical block techniques and books which should be published by experienced users.

Nevertheless, close supervision for those who intend to start with this technique should be part of an educational framework. In recent years, the number of practical users has constantly grown, resulting in great improvements across the field. In addition, guidelines for the adequate use of ultrasound-guided regional anaesthesia and recommendations on how to start are now available; these should serve as a basic introduction to the technique.

Figure 4.3 provides a suggestion for a training concept in 'Ultrasound-guided regional anaesthesia'. The time frame from the initial basic workshop to a masterclass workshop can be estimated to one and a half years. Those who have passed a masterclass workshop should be able to perform all levels of ultrasound-guided regional anaesthesia blocks in a safe and highly effective manner.

The large regional anaesthesia societies (European Society of Regional Anaesthesia and Pain Therapy (ESRA) and American Society of Regional Anaesthesia and Pain Medicine (ASRA)) have recently published initial recommendations for education and training in ultrasound-guided regional anaesthesia. Anyway, it will still be a long way from dedicated theoretical considerations to a broad acceptance and the subsequent practical implementation.

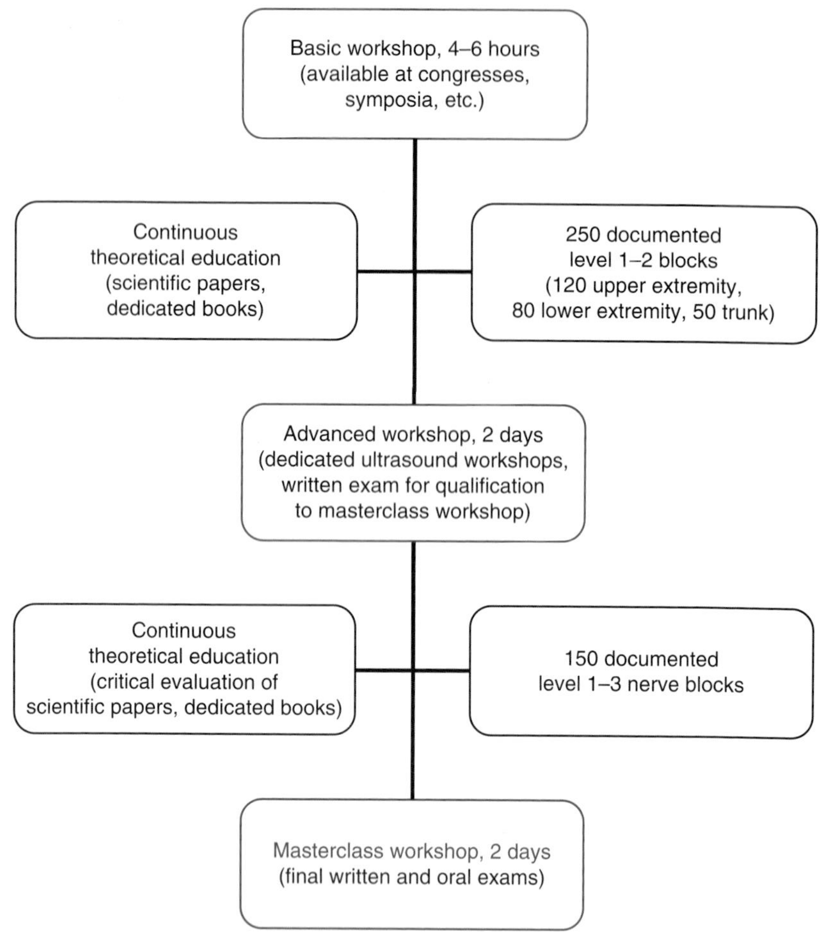

Fig. 4.3 Suggested concept for appropriate education in 'Ultrasound-guided regional anaesthesia'. This algorithm is not scientifically evaluated, but should serve as a rough concept to achieve a masterclass level, where blocks of all difficulties can be managed.

Suggested further reading

Ivani, G., Ferrante, F.M., 2009. The American Society of Regional Anaesthesia and Pain Medicine and the European Society of Regional Anaesthesia and Pain Therapy Joint Committee recommendations for education and training in ultrasound-guided regional anaesthesia: why do we need these guidelines? *Regional Anesthesia and Pain Medicine*, 34(1), pp.8–9.

Sites, B.D., Chan, V.W., Neal, J.M., Weller, R., Grau, T., Koscielniak–Nielsen, Z.J., Ivani, G., 2009. The American Society of Regional Anaesthesia and Pain Medicine and the European Society of Regional Anaesthesia and Pain Therapy Joint Committee recommendations for education and training in ultrasound-guided regional anaesthesia. *Regional Anesthesia and Pain Medicine*, 34(1), pp.40–6.

Chapter 5

Have we reached the gold standard in regional anaesthesia?

Regional anaesthesia is a 'simple' specialty. It just requires that the right dose of the right drug is administered at the right place. Therefore, the direct visualization of neuronal structures, the adjacent anatomy, and the spread of local anaesthetic must be beneficial to achieve optimal block success and avoid complications. Anyway, in order to optimize the performance of ultrasound-guided regional block techniques, some key points should be discussed.

Much has been speculated and discussed about the optimal site of administration of the local anaesthetic. An extra-epineural needle position is safe and effective from today's point of view whereas the perineural position of the needle is controversial. Despite the fact that there is limited evidence to support one of the two puncture techniques, theoretical considerations favour the technique where the local anaesthetic is administered around the nerve structure. The possibility of neuronal damage due to a local anaesthetic-induced high pressure during perineural administration is one concern against this technique. Additionally, despite the high ultrasound frequencies nowadays, an intraneural position of the needle tip can never be excluded once the epineurium is pierced to perform an intra-epineural technique.

Another important topic is the volume of local anaesthetic necessary to provide a successful nerve block. It is a matter of fact that large volumes of local anaesthetic have been used in the past to compensate for inexact techniques of nerve identification. Despite these inappropriate large volumes at times, the success rates of various regional techniques were rather disappointing. The most likely reason for such weak success rates is the inexact identification of nerve structures. Recent studies indicate that peripheral nerve blocks can be performed with much lower volumes of local anaesthetic as described in the past. Eichenberger et al. shows that successful ultrasonographic-guided ulnar nerve blockade is possible with less than 1mL of local anaesthetic. The authors of that study used an up-and-down statistical study design and a novel method to calculate the particular volume of local anaesthetic based on the individual cross-sectional nerve area. Thus, a reliable evaluation of the effective dose $(ED)_{95}$ of 0.11mL/mm^2 cross-sectional nerve area for this particular nerve block was possible. Similar results as presented by Eichenberger et al. for an upper extremity nerve has been shown by Latzke et al. for the sciatic nerve blockade, where the ED_{99} was determined with 0.10mL/mm^2 cross-sectional nerve area. The median cross-sectional nerve area was 57mm^2 in that volunteer study, resulting in a median volume of 5.7mL of local anaesthetic for sciatic nerve blockade. The lowest volume for a successful sciatic nerve blockade in that study was 1.7mL. Figure 5.1 shows this case where a complete surrounding of the nerve with local anaesthetic was not achieved. Thus, a re-evaluation of the concept that the local anaesthetic has to surround the entire nerve for a successful blockade ('donut sign') seems to be necessary.

It is important to mention that such low-volume blocks can only be realized with a multi-injection technique, even for single nerve blocks. For more sophisticated techniques such as interscalene or axillary brachial plexus blocks, various particular needle tip positions are required to realize a successful low-volume block. In fact, the spread of local anaesthetic during a particular needle tip position can never be predicted and therefore, an immediate adjustment of the needle tip position following every injection is a prerequisite for the realization of this technique.

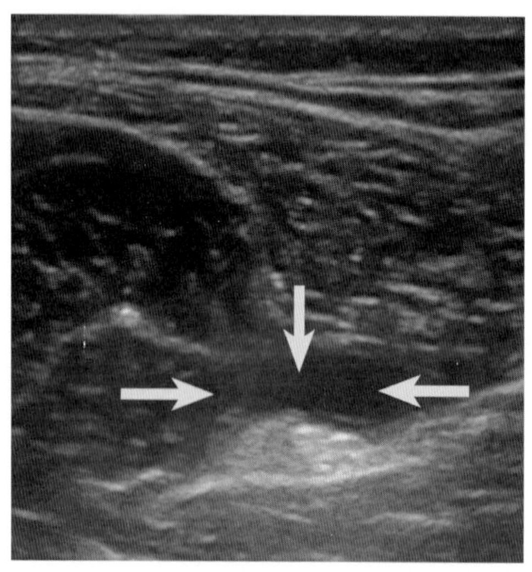

Fig. 5.1 Ultrasound illustration of the sciatic nerve at the mid-femoral level, where the local anaesthetic does not completely surround the nerve. The arrows indicate the hypoechoic local anaesthetic solution.

It seems that we are on a good way to achieve a level where we can talk about a 'gold standard' in regional anaesthesia. Anyway, it is important to highlight limitations why the final target—that is optimal block success, no complications or relevant side effects—is still not always reached. The main reason for this is the fact that there are simply too many descriptions for particular scanning or block techniques available. The scientific value of case reports or small observational studies is limited, leading more to confusion than to an increase in knowledge and improvement of hand skills. Thus, the quality of science is still not optimal and there is a lot of room for improvement. The scientific quality of ultrasound in regional anaesthesia is closely associated with the broad use of the technique in daily clinical practice. To reach a 'gold standard' in a particular technique requires both excellent science and the responsible and careful implementation in clinical practice. Retrospectively, we have never reached a 'gold standard' in regional anaesthesia. Techniques with an average success rate of 80% cannot be described as 'gold standard'. The use of ultrasound for regional blocks may provide for the first time the establishment of any 'standard' in this subspecialty if a responsible and careful implementation of the technique is performed.

The topic of patient's satisfaction is closely associated with these areas of great importance. Our patients will decide if a technique achieves all criteria required to be considered as 'gold standard'. Patients should be satisfied with an anaesthetic technique which provides a predictable and pain-free experience of their surgical procedure. But anaesthetists (like other physicians) tend to overestimate their own performance and therefore, a scientific evaluation of this topic is also absolutely required.

But the best technique lacks any value without a global spread. More than a billion human beings have no access to modern medicine. The lack of anaesthesia needed for surgery is one of the main problems in this context. Ultrasound for regional blocks could provide a significant input for various surgical procedures in remote areas or where the economical situation is disastrous. Thus, the opinion leaders in this field and companies and governments of first and second world countries are requested to find adequate solutions to this situation. Clearly, the eradication of malaria is more popular than the broad use of regional anaesthesia for surgery, but pain-free surgical procedures should be a human right. The development of basic and subsequently cheap ultrasound equipment for this specific use, similar to that of basic laptop computers for third world countries, would be a prerequisite for the implementation of ultrasound for regional blocks all over the world. The 'gold standard' in regional anaesthesia is only achieved when this most important target has been realized.

In summary, a 'gold standard' in regional anaesthesia should be defined as follows:

1 Adequate scientific descriptions of all aspects in that field.
2 Administration of local anaesthetic around the nerve as close as possible to the nerve structure(s) with an extra-epineural needle position.
3 Multi-injection technique.
4 Use of optimal volumes of the local anaesthetic.
5 Success rate above 98%.
6 No complication due to the puncture technique.
7 Global practical use of the particular techniques.

Chapter 6

Technical and organization prerequisites for ultrasonographic-guided blocks

Some important issues should be considered prior to the introduction of ultrasound-guided regional anaesthesia in daily clinical practice. It is of particular importance to highlight the necessity of considering technical and organizational requirements for the adequate and optimal use of this technique and its initial introduction.

6.1 Technical considerations

6.1.1 Optimal equipment

Every institution and individual physician should carefully decide which ultrasound equipment is optimal for their purposes. Since the advent of portable equipment, ultrasound machines have become much more affordable and, due to intensive research, the image quality of portable machines is now similar to larger and more expensive ones. The quality of 2D imaging has improved due to frequency compounding procedures and subsequent speckle noise reduction. The frame rate of 2D imaging during colour Doppler is also now increased with the effect of equal image quality as compared with the pure 2D mode.

Nevertheless, the initial costs for ultrasound equipment are significant, even for relatively low-priced machines. It is therefore necessary to calculate the overall costs for this new and innovative technique, taking into consideration aspects of the individual institution.

Due to the enormous interest in ultrasound-guided regional anaesthesia, some manufacturers have designed specialized equipment adapted specifically for the purposes of visualization of nerves. We have found that it is cost-effective to avoid non-specific software and/or tools and to focus on one specific indication. In cases where a machine is shared with other subspecialties (e.g. intensive care), additional software might be useful. All in all, additional costs should not be an insurmountable problem in providing optimal care for our patients.

6.1.2 Which probes are appropriate?

All superficial block techniques can be performed with multifrequent linear ultrasound probes. Today's technology allows frequencies up to 15MHz, where even maximal superficial nerve structures are visible. Higher frequencies are not useful because of reduced penetration depth. An ultrasound probe with a frequency of 20MHz allows a penetration depth of only 1–1.25cm and is therefore of limited practical use. Regional techniques where the nerves are deeper (e.g. psoas compartment, anterior approach to the sciatic nerve) should be performed with lower frequent sector probes.

6.1.3 Needle equipment

The appropriate ultrasonographic visibility of needles is an important consideration. Several manufacturers have designed needles specifically for ultrasound purposes by using different materials or surfaces. No needle has yet been shown in a scientific way to have a particular advantage over other needles. In fact, the better the visibility of a needle, the more image artefacts are caused.

Maecken et al. (2007) investigated the ultrasound visibility of different needles in two media (water bath and animal model) with three different ultrasound machines and two angles (0° and 45°). The authors of this observational study found differences in the visibility of the needles and defined the following requirements for the 'ideal needle':

- Good needle visibility, in particular the needle tip.
- Suitability for all kinds of tissue.
- Good visualization at all angles.
- Sharp depiction of the needle rim.
- Low artefact formation.
- No shadowing.
- Extremely good detection and differentiation from the surrounding area.

No studies are available that investigate the success rates with different needle types. In other words, we have no information if the 'ideal needle', which does not exist from today's point of view, improves success rate and safety.

Piezoelectric vibrating needles are one example of recent developments, where colour-flow Doppler is used to identify the tip of the needle. Two piezoelectric actuators use this technology to create 1–8kHz vibrations, thus facilitating the identification of the tip of the needle (Figure 6.1). Another promising technology to improve the detection of the tip of the needle and to predict the path of the needle is the use of a GPS equivalent (Figure 6.2).

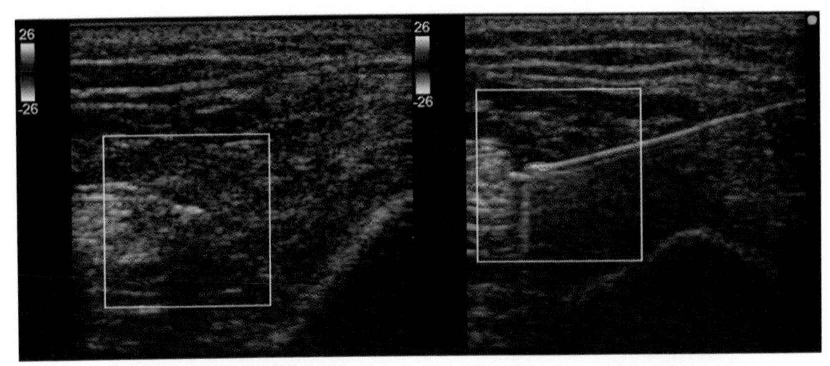

Fig. 6.1 Ultrasound illustration of a piezoelectric needle during the OOP (left) and IP (right) needle guidance techniques.

An *injection line* is useful for all types of needles in order to realize an 'immobile needle technique' according to Winnie (1969) (Figures 6.3 and 6.4). A technique where the syringe is directly connected to the needle is associated with inadvertent needle movement and is therefore inexact and should be avoided.

Figures 6.5 to 6.9 illustrate specific ultrasound and non-specific ultrasound needle equipment from various manufacturers. An estimation of the relative ultrasound visibility of needles is possible by evaluating the differences in histogram values between the tip and body of the needle and the surrounding tissue. One program where these measurements can be performed is Adobe Photoshop (Adobe™ Inc., San Jose, USA). Table 5 provides measurements

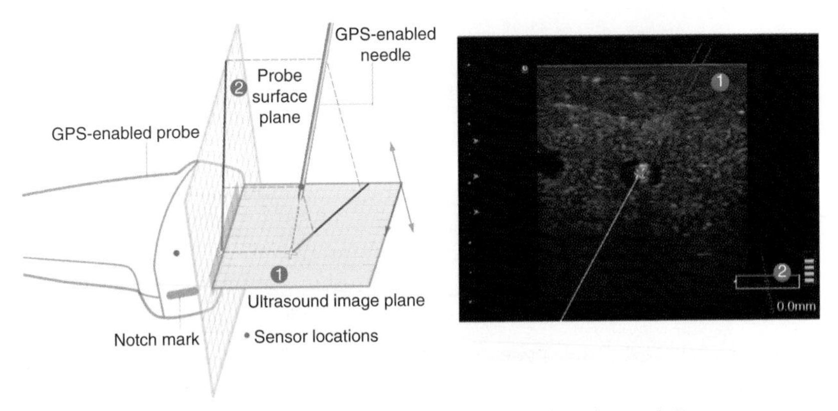

Fig. 6.2 GPS-like needle guidance technology, provided by Ultrasonix™.

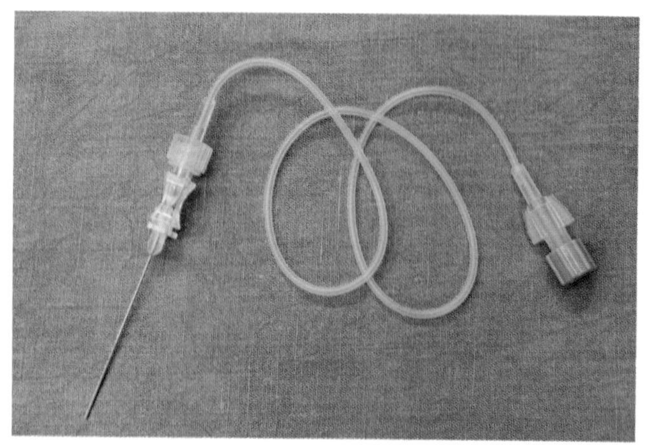

Fig. 6.3 Needle with injection line (22G, Facette tip).

where the differences of specific histograms (measured area is 100 pixel) of the following areas were evaluated:

- Tip of the needle–surrounding tissue (IP 10° and 45°).
- Body of the needle–surrounding tissue (IP 10° and 45°).
- Tip of the needle–surrounding tissue (OOP 5mm and 15mm deep).

The six measurements can be added and the mean score allows an estimation regarding needle visibility, where a low number indicates lower ultrasound visibility and a high number indicates a good visibility. It is important

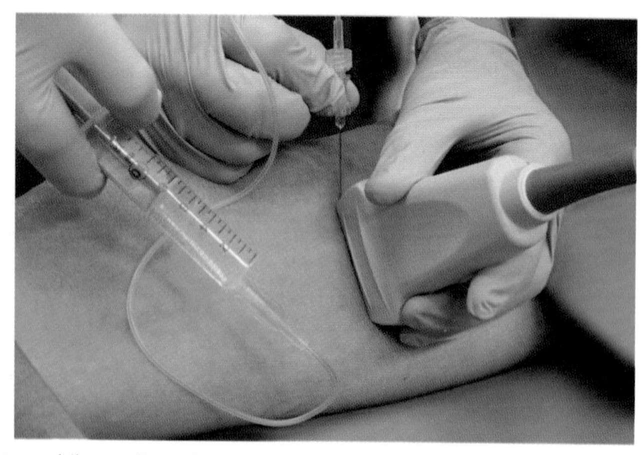

Fig. 6.4 Immobile needle technique where the syringe is connected with an injection line.

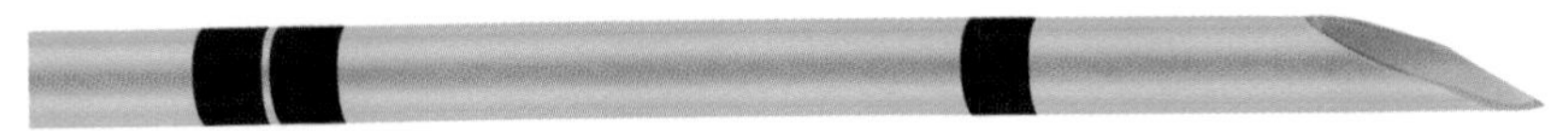

Fig. 6.5 Peripheral nerve block needle with Facette tip.

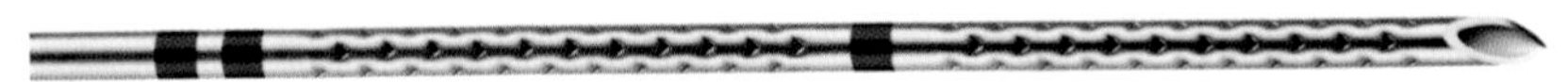

Fig. 6.6 Peripheral nerve block needle with Facette tip and a particular echogenic surface.

Fig. 6.7 Peripheral nerve block needle with a Sprotte tip.

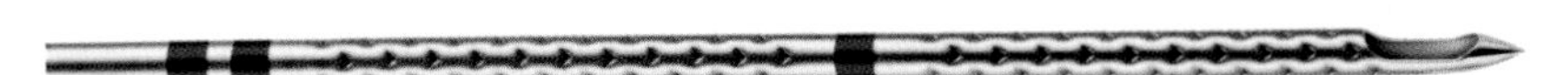

Fig. 6.8 Peripheral nerve block needle with a Sprotte tip and a particular echogenic surface.

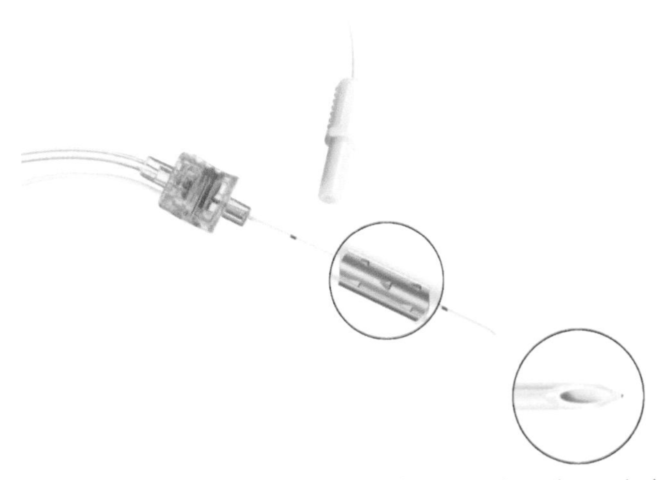

Fig. 6.9 Peripheral isolated nerve block needle with Facette tip and a particular echogenic surface.

Table 5 Mean histogram values (evaluated in Adobe Photoshop CS3, Adobe™ Inc., San Jose, USA) of different needles. The measurements have been evaluated with a 38 mm 13MHz linear ultrasound probe in fascial free meat. The histogram values are based on averages after 5 measurements

Needle description	Size	Tip	Isolation	Orientation	Histogram values needle tip, surounding tissue and difference			Histogram values needle body, surounding tissue and difference			Mean histogram score: needle tip	Mean histogram score: needle body	Total histogram score
Polymedic 'Ultrasound needle'	21G	Facette	No	IP 10°	132	14	118	70	14	56	98	31	76
				IP 45°	123	14	109	20	14	6			
				OOP 5mm	76	14	62						
				OOP 15mm	118	15	103						
Pajunk 'Sonoplex'	21G	Facette	No	IP 10°	130	15	115	57	13	44	82	47	70
				IP 45°	66	7	59	60	11	49			
				OOP 5mm	105	15	90						
				OOP 15mm	80	15	65						
Pajunk 'Uniplex'	25G	Facette	No	IP 10°	103	10	93	99	13	86	80	46	68
				IP 45°	78	8	70	22	16	6			
				OOP 5mm	78	14	64						
				OOP 15mm	101	10	91						
Pajunk 'Uniplex nanoline'	22G	Facette	No	IP 10°	97	13	84	74	14	60	84	33	67
				IP 45°	102	11	91	15	10	5			
				OOP 5mm	70	10	60						
				OOP 15mm	111	9	102						
Pajunk 'Sonoplex'	22G	Facette	No	IP 10°	74	16	58	82	18	64	63	66	64
				IP 45°	70	13	57	84	16	68			
				OOP 5mm	54	11	43						
				OOP 15mm	107	14	93						
Pajunk 'Uniplex nanoline'	22G	Sprotte	No	IP 10°	78	13	65	106	8	98	61	55	59
				IP 45°	77	12	65	20	9	11			
				OOP 5mm	50	8	42						
				OOP 15mm	84	13	71						

Pajunk 'Uniplex'	22G	Sprotte	No	IP 10°	70	18	52	73	6	67	65	37	56
				IP 45°	97	17	80	19	13	6			
				OOP 5mm	70	6	64						
				OOP 15mm	83	18	65						
BBraun 'Stimuplex D'	25G	15°	Yes	IP 10°	67	7	60	49	7	42	64	23	50
				IP 45°	64	9	55	13	10	3			
				OOP 5mm	71	6	65						
				OOP 15mm	89	12	77						
Pajunk 'Epidural'	18G	Tuohy	no	IP 10°	60	12	48	53	7	46	61	29	50
				IP 45°	110	11	99	24	12	12			
				OOP 5mm	67	13	54						
				OOP 15mm	62	20	42						
BBraun 'Stimuplex D Plus'	22G	15°	Yes	IP 10°	67	12	55	61	16	45	54	26	44
				IP 45°	77	15	62	12	6	6			
				OOP 5mm	48	13	35						
				OOP 15mm	82	20	62						
Pajunk 'Spinal'	27G	Sprotte	No	IP 10°	67	11	56	51	8	43	53	24	43
				IP 45°	80	14	66	16	12	4			
				OOP 5mm	49	14	35						
				OOP 15mm	71	17	54						
BBraun 'Stimuplex D'	22G	30°	Yes	IP 10°	67	12	64	63	14	49	46	25	39
				IP 45°	30	14	16	10	10	0			
				OOP 5mm	56	11	45						
				OOP 15mm	75	16	59						
BBraun 'Stimuplex A'	21G	30°	No	IP 10°	68	13	55	53	6	47	39	24	34
				IP 45°	33	12	21	20	19	1			
				OOP 5mm	53	10	43						
				OOP 15mm	56	19	37						

to state that this method is not scientifically evaluated, but nevertheless useful to estimate grey scales.

According to the measurements illustrated in Table 5, the subsequent rules can be stated regarding ultrasound visibility of different needles.

Diameter of the needle

The needle size has only minor influence on needle visibility. Exact guidance technique is therefore more important for needle visibility (Figure 6.10).

Angle of insertion

A flat angle of insertion provides better visualization when an IP technique is used whereas a steep angle of insertion causes impaired needle visualization (Figure 6.11). Recent developments in needle visibility allow improved needle visibility for steeper angles as well (Figure 6.12). For the OOP technique, steeper angles of insertion are associated with a tendency of better visualization of the needle tip (Figure 6.13).

Tip of the needle

The different shapes of needle tips do not significantly influence ultrasound visualization (Figure 6.14). The differences of needle tips affect mainly clinical features, such as pain during needle insertion (facette tip needles are associated with less pain than Tuohy needle tips) and the possibility of accurate needle placement ('sharp' needle tips allow a more accurate needle tip placement than blunt needle tips).

In summary, there is currently no scientific evidence for significant advantages of so-called 'ultrasound needles'. There is a tendency for improved qualities of visibility in some aspects (e.g. IP steeper angles), but the entire topic is extremely complex and any simplification may lead to wrong interpretations. The individual hand skills are of utmost importance in this context. Nevertheless, the use of ultrasound products in daily clinical practice has been found to be cost-effective. The avoidance of using an electric cable for nerve stimulation purposes and an isolated shaft may significantly lower costs once these needles are produced in large numbers.

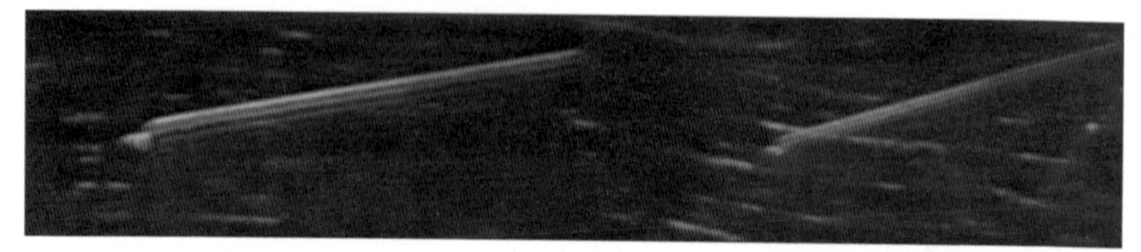

Fig. 6.10 IP needle guidance technique to illustrate the similar echogenicity of a 21G (left) vs a 25G (right) Facette tip needle.Technique performed in a psoas major pork muscle.

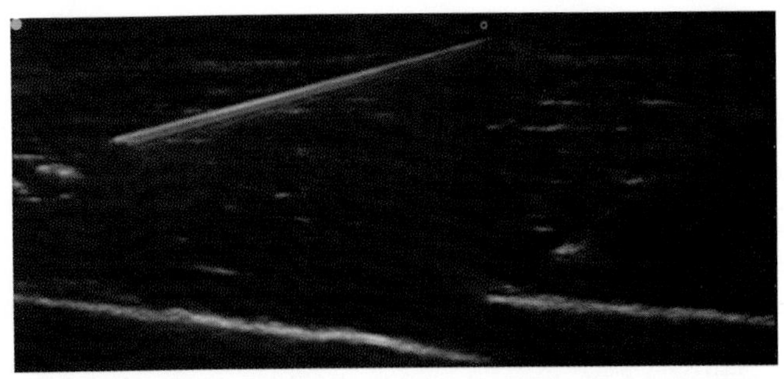

Fig. 6.11 IP needle guidance technique to illustrate the better needle visibility of a flat vs a steep angle.Technique performed in a psoas major pork muscle.

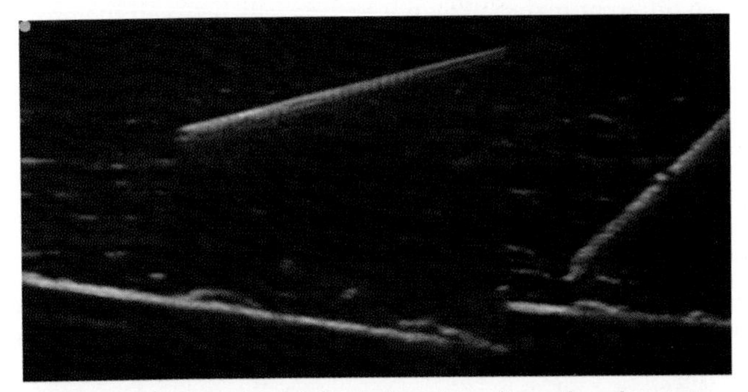

Fig. 6.12 Improved visibility of specially designed needle surface for steep angles.

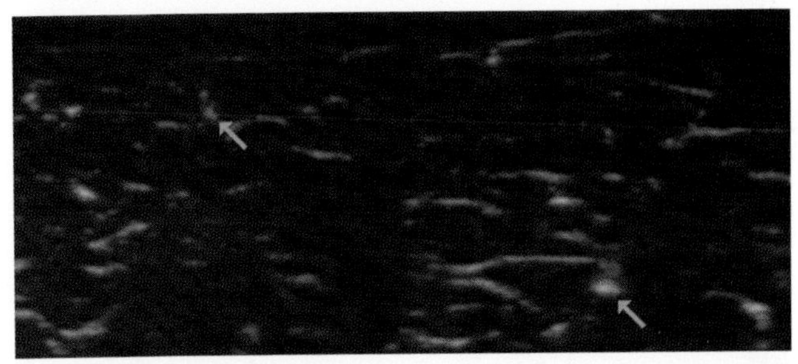

Fig. 6.13 OOP needle guidance technique to illustrate the needle tip visibility of superficial vs deeper needle tip position.The deep needle tip position (left) provides improved visibility of the needle tip visibility compared with the more superficial needle tip position (right).

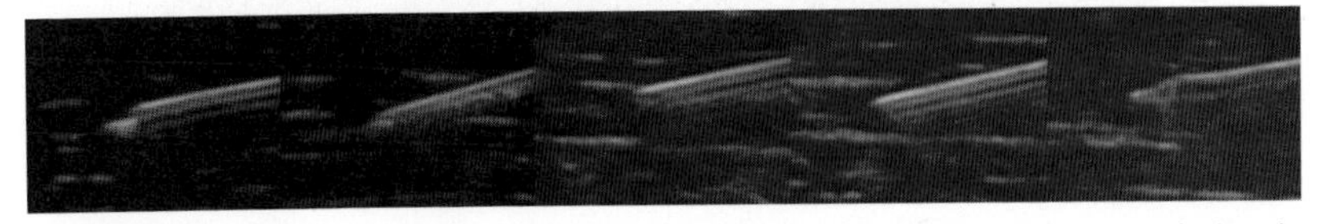

Fig. 6.14 Ultrasound visibility of different needle tips (IP needle guidance technique). From left to right: Facette, Sprotte, 15°, 30°, Tuohy.

6.1.4 Sterility

Sterile preparation of the probe and block area is a prerequisite for ultrasound-guided block techniques. Subspecialties such as interventional radiology have been using covered probes for many years in order to preserve sterility. Despite their extensive experience with ultrasound-guided interventions, an optimal cover has yet to be identified.

The expert statement paper published in 2007 (see Appendix 1 for a summary) recommends a sterile probe cover for single and continuous block techniques. Figure 6.15 shows the latest development in that field, where a transparent adhesive sheet is connected to a plastic foil. This unique arrangement of two different materials avoids getting jelly between the probe and the cover. Of course, (sterile) jelly between the probe cover and the skin is necessary. We have found that urinary catheter jelly can be used as an alternative to dedicated and more expensive sterile ultrasound products. Figures 6.16 to 6.19 illustrate how the sterile ultrasound probe cover should be used.

Figures 6.20 and 6.21 compare the histogram values of an ultrasound illustration (psoas major muscle of a pig, two different gain adjustments) of a 13MHz linear probe without probe cover, with a glove as probe cover and two jelly layers, and with a specific ultrasound probe cover with one jelly layer. The probe without cover provides the brightest image quality, whereas

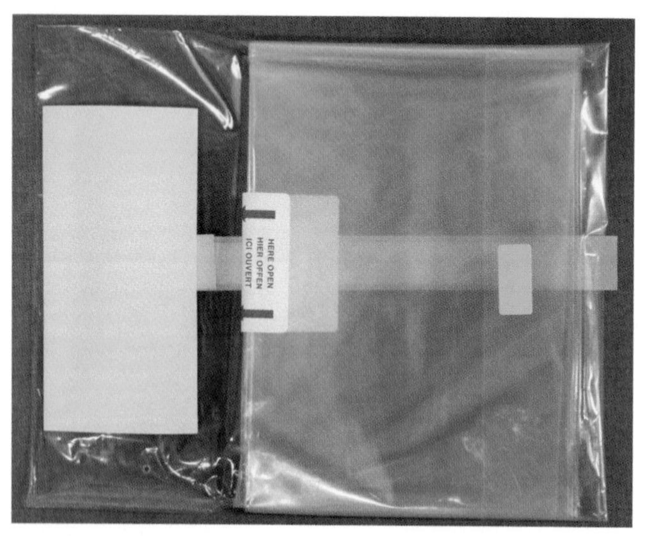

Fig. 6.15 Sterile probe cover system with a transparent adhesive sheet (left side) which is connected to a plastic foil.

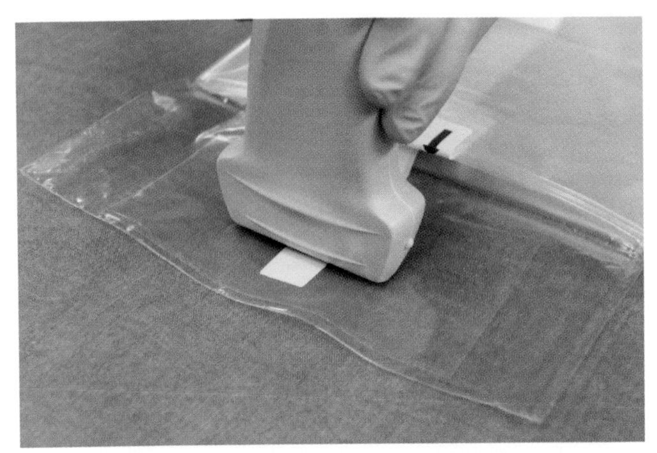

Fig. 6.16 Correct use of the sterile probe cover.The active area of this linear probe is placed on the adhesive part of the probe cover.

the images of the probe with the glove and the specific ultrasound probe cover appear slightly darker. Thus, the use of probe covers requires slight adjustments in gain to compensate for the loss of brightness (+4% 'glove cover' and +7% 'specific ultrasound probe cover' as compared with 'no probe cover').

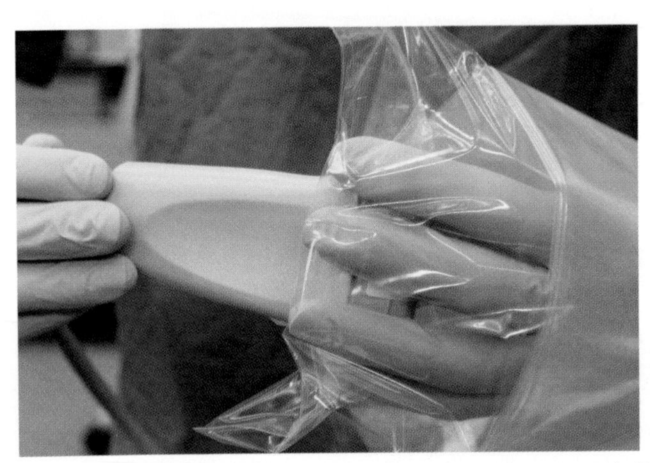

Fig. 6.17 Correct use of the sterile probe cover.The probe is then covered all over by the plastic sheath.

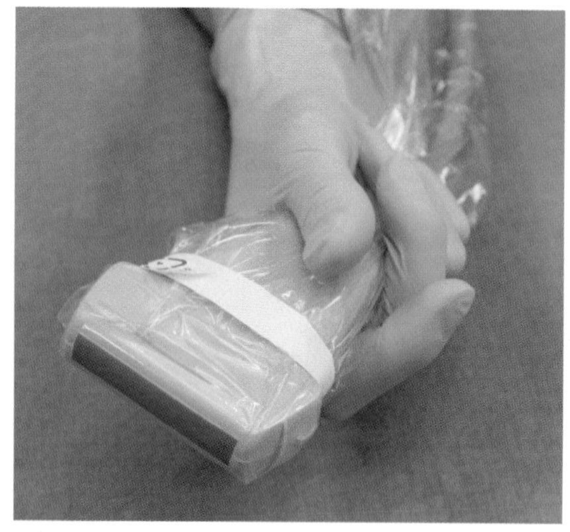

Fig. 6.18 The ultrasound probe and the cable are covered in a sterile manner.

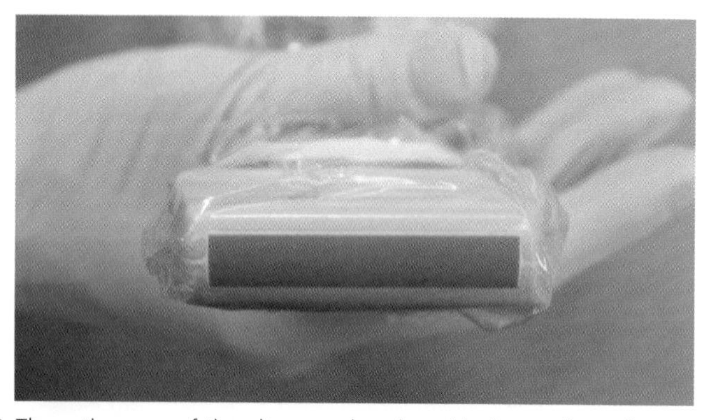

Fig. 6.19 The active area of the ultrasound probe with the sterile probe cover. It is important to avoid any creases in order to maintain optimal image quality which is easily possible with this system.

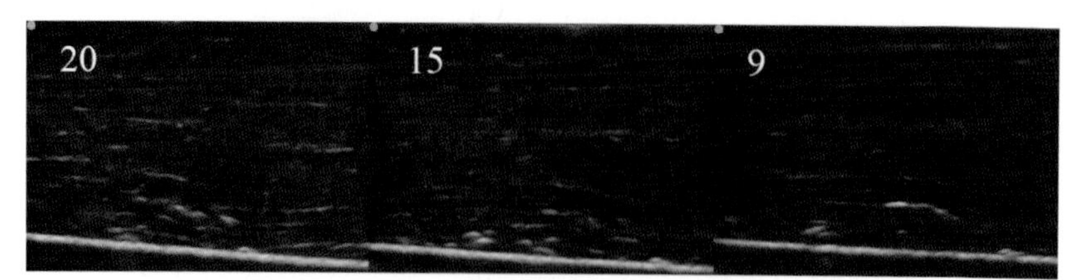

Fig. 6.20 Histogram values of a 13MHz linear probe without probe cover (left), with a glove as probe cover and two jelly layers (middle), and with a specific ultrasound probe cover with one jelly layer (right). The numbers indicate the specific histogram values from the entire screen shot (approx. 100,000 pixels for each screen shot).

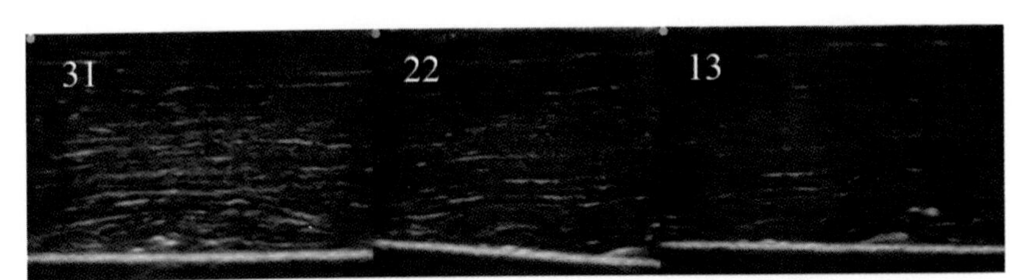

Fig. 6.21 Histogram values of a 13MHz linear probe without probe cover (left), with a glove as probe cover and two jelly layers (middle), and with a specific ultrasound probe cover with one jelly layer (right). The numbers indicate the specific histogram values from the entire screen shot (approx. 100,000 pixels for each screen shot). Different gain adjustment as in Figure 6.20.

6.2 **Organization**

6.2.1 **How to start?**

Adequate education and training is necessary to achieve the courageous aim of successful ultrasound-guided regional blocks. All anaesthesia congresses provide basic workshops aiming at stimulating the interest of potential users of this technique. These very basic workshops should be followed by advanced and expert workshops. Anyway, the anaesthesia community is at a very early stage in the development of guidelines for a structured education. Chapter 4 provides a concept of appropriate training and education in ultrasound-guided regional anaesthesia.

Once the institution of an individual physician is willing to implement ultrasound guidance in their regional, clinical, anaesthetic practice, the following questions should be clearly answered:

- How was their own performance of regional anaesthesia in terms of overall success rates and complications in the past?
- Is there room for improvement when the technique of nerve guidance will be changed?
- What prerequisites should be considered when ultrasound guidance for regional blocks will be introduced?
- How can we monitor problems associated with the new technique?
- How can we review our daily clinical practice?
- How can we avoid problems which are inherent to the system?

A critical self-reflection is necessary to provide honest answers to all these questions. A structured concept of training and education in ultrasound-guided regional anaesthesia is helpful to change clinical practice, but the initial intention for a change in clinical practice must come from the individual practitioner.

6.2.2 Where should the blocks be performed?

Whether regional nerve blocks are performed in or out of the operating room (OR) depends on the internal organization of the institutions. In our experience with both locations, we have found that the advantage of a dedicated 'block room' is that it can be adapted to suit the specific purposes of regional blocks. After nerve blockade, the patient can be transported into the OR and the surgical procedure can start without delay, thus resulting in a smooth OR process. Giving proper consideration to the onset and duration of the blockade allows for a more efficient time management.

6.3 Post-operative observation

Optimal patient care also includes post-anaesthesia care. In our experience over the past decade, we have observed that ultrasound-guided block techniques reduce the length of stay in the post-anaesthesia care unit. Due to improved block qualities in comparison with conventional techniques as well as extremely low conversion rates to general anaesthetic techniques, most patients can bypass the post-anaesthesia care unit altogether. Patients can be transferred straight to the ward or even directly discharged home, which is cost-effective and improves patient comfort.

6.4 Other considerations

6.4.1 Monitoring

Minimal requirements for monitoring during the performance of ultrasound-guided blocks are:

- Intravenous line
- Pulse oximetry
- Electrocardiogram
- Blood pressure monitoring.

Depending on the medical status of the patient and the surgical procedure, additional monitoring might be necessary.

6.4.2 Management of emergencies

Serious side effects during regional blocks are extremely rare, but should be managed appropriately once such an event occurs. There is no evidence that ultrasound has the potency to completely eliminate serious side effects such as a rapid increase of local anaesthetic blood levels. Thus, facilities for cardiopulmonary resuscitation should be available wherever regional techniques are performed. Appendix 3 provides the current guidelines for lipid resuscitation for the management of local anaesthetic intoxication.

Suggested further reading

Maecken, T., Zenz, M., Grau, T., 2007. Ultrasound characteristics of needles for regional anaesthesia. *Regional Anaesthesia and Pain Medicine*, 32(5), pp.440–7.

Winnie, A.P., 1969. An 'immobile needle' for nerve blocks. *Anesthesiology*, 31(6), 577–8.

Chapter 7

Ultrasound-guided regional anaesthetic techniques in children: current developments and particular considerations

The interest of various regional techniques in paediatric anaesthesia is increasing. Ultrasound may contribute to increasing the safety and effectiveness of paediatric regional anaesthesia in daily clinical practice. However, a lot of efforts in terms of training, acquiring hand skills, and modification of operation processes are required to implement ultrasound-guided paediatric techniques in daily clinical practice. The highly sophisticated regional anaesthetic techniques and subsequent alterations in general anaesthesia management may lead directly to discussions referring to dedicated specialists in the field of paediatric anaesthesia.

A systematic review regarding the efficacy and safety of ultrasound-guided peripheral and central blocks in children described that only three clinical studies achieved an adequate scientific level (Table 6), whereas six publications were identified as sufficient in answering the question if ultrasound shows advantages for neuraxial blocks (Table 7). Ilioinguinal-iliohypogastric nerve blocks and epidural catheterization are well described in the literature whereas exact descriptions of blocks of the upper and lower extremities are still lacking.

In general, ultrasound-guided blocks in children are easier compared with techniques in adults. Most anatomical structures are superficial and therefore easier to detect by high-frequency ultrasound. Thus, high-frequency linear ultrasound probes are appropriate for most block techniques in children. In smaller children, ultrasound probes with smaller surfaces are more suitable.

For peripheral nerve blocks, most techniques may be performed with 22G facette tip needles. In children less than 3 years old and for very superficial blocks, 24G facette tip needles can be considered. For epidural blockade, appropriate Tuohy needles and (if indicated) catheters should be considered. The suggested needle sizes are described in Chapter 16, Section 16.4.1.

Table 6 Randomized controlled studies on ultrasound-guided peripheral regional techniques in children*

Publication	Technique	Study design and significant outcome
Marhofer et al. (*Anaesthesia*, 2004)	Infraclavicular brachial plexus block	Comparison with nerve stimulation: faster sensory and motor onset times, longer duration of block, less pain during performance of the block when ultrasound was used
Oberndorfer et al. (*British Journal of Anaesthesia*, 2007)	Sciatic and femoral nerve blocks	Comparison with nerve stimulation: longer duration of sensory block and smaller volumes of local anaesthetic when ultrasound was used
Willschke et al. (*British Journal of Anaesthesia*, 2005)	Ilioinguinal-iliohypogastric nerve blocks	Comparison with 'fascial click': less intraoperative and post-operative requirements for additional analgesia, smaller volumes of local anaesthetic when ultrasound was used

* Rubin et al. (2009)

For local anaesthetics, less concentrated drugs can be used in smaller children due to incomplete myelin sheets of peripheral nerves. Whenever possible, post-operative motor block should be avoided to increase the comfort of our little patients. As for all ultrasound-guided regional techniques, the volumes of local anaesthetics can be reduced as compared with non-ultrasound-guided techniques. Recommendations for volumes of local anaesthetics are included wherever relevant in the following chapters.

7.1 Management of minor trauma in children

Most of the minor trauma cases in children are equitable with broken legs. Unfortunately, it is still a worldwide used practice that repositioning of fractured legs is performed without any analgesic treatment or with the administration of local anaesthetic in between the fracture. Thus, management of children undergoing extremity surgery following trauma can be effectively performed by ultrasound-guided blocks of the brachial or lumbosacral plexus.

Most techniques in adult clinical practice can also be used for children. Technical characteristics specific for upper and lower limb blocks are described in Chapters 13 and 14. The main difference between adults and children is the *miscellaneous management* (informed consent, sedation, etc.). In most cases, children do not show any insight into their illness and therefore, some additional general anaesthesia management is required. In any case, a direct

Table 7 Randomized controlled studies regarding ultrasound-guided neuraxial regional techniques in children*

Publication	Technique	Study design and significant outcome
Chawathe et al. (*Pediatric Anesthesia*, 2003)	Observation of epidural catheter	Case series: visualization of the epidural catheter was possible in 9 in 12 children, all of these aged under 6 months
Roberts et al. (*Pediatric Anesthesia*, 2005)	Assessment of the position of caudal catheters	Case series: visualization of the tip of the caudal catheter at a thoracic level was possible in 1 in 3 infants
Rapp et al. (*Anesthesia & Analgesia*, 2005)	Ultrasound-assisted epidural catheter insertion	Case series: identification of neuraxial structures with ultrasonography, identification of epidural catheter in 11 in 23 cases
Willschke et al. (*British Journal of Anaesthesia*, 2006)	Ultrasound-assisted epidural catheter placement	Randomized, controlled trial: swifter performance of epidural catheter placement when ultrasound was used when compared with the conventional loss-of-resistance technique, observation of the spread of local anaesthetic in the epidural space with ultrasound
Willschke et al. (*Regional Anesthesia and Pain Medicine*, 2007)	Ultrasound-assisted epidural catheter placement	Evaluation of the neuraxial sonoanatomy in neonates. Correlation of the depth of the flavum ligament by ultrasound and needle insertion depth with the loss-of-resistance technique; case series of ultrasound-assisted epidural catheter placement in neonates and infants under 4kg: ultrasound provides significant information during epidural catheter placement in neonates and infants
Kil et al. (*Regional Anesthesia and Pain Medicine*, 2007)	Ultrasound-assisted epidural catheter placement	Prepuncture measurement of the depth of the flavum ligament: information on the depth of the flavum ligament increases the margin of safety during epidural catheter placement

* Rubin et al. (2009)

approach and attention to the child is useful and possible in most cases. Depending on their social and intellectual competences, children are able to communicate in an appropriate manner from the age of 4 years. In other words, communication between the physician and the patient is one of the most important prerequisites for an appropriate treatment of these paediatric cases.

The role of the parents is also important in this context. Parents should always feel that they are fully informed and involved in the treatment of their children and therefore, an open communication is necessary to build a mutual trust. Usually parents expect some kind of 'general anaesthesia' when their children are admitted to hospital due to an accident. After more than a decade treating these children, I cannot remember one case where the parents did not agree with the performance of a regional anaesthetic technique. Due to the fact that we treat a multinational collective of patients, we are able to suggest this kind of treatment for a large variety of nations.

Figure 7.1 shows an algorithm for sedation of children with broken legs. The algorithm indicates that children under severe pain are treated faster than children with no or moderate pain. Most of the time during the treatment of this patient population can be saved by omitting the use of EMLA cream for the venous and regional anaesthesia puncture site. In cases of severe pain caused by the injury, every method of premedication seems to be impractical and inappropriate due to time consumption. In other words, the management of minor trauma of extremities in children depends on the status of pain:

- Severe pain: maximal reduction of the time from admission to block.
- Mild to moderate pain: the comfort of pain reduction by using EMLA cream can be considered prior to the insertion of a venous access and at the possible puncture site of the regional anaesthetic technique. An initial investigation of the possible regional anaesthetic puncture site is useful in detecting anatomical reasons for alternative approaches and to avoid unnecessary drug exposure with EMLA cream.

The method of sedation is highly individual. Our current practice is based on a combination of iv midazolam (0.05–0.1mg/kg), iv nalbuphine (0.1mg/kg), and iv propofol (0.5–2mg/kg). It is important to consider that drug effects (even if only minor) in paediatric trauma cases are highly individual and therefore, the doses above serve only as a rough indication. Depending on the individual, internal, institutional guidelines for paediatric sedation, a large variety of drugs can be used and we recommend that physicians should use familiar drugs. There is no need to change the institutional paediatric sedation protocol for regional anaesthesia purposes.

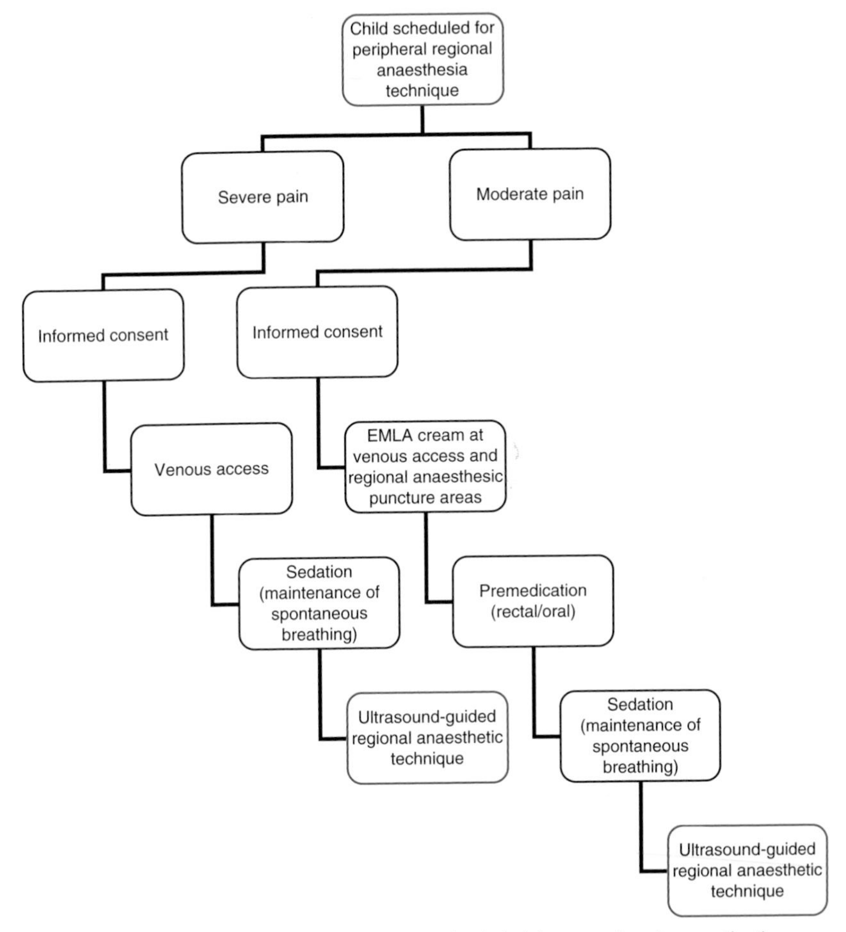

Fig. 7.1 Algorithm for sedation in children scheduled for a regional anaesthetic technique following minor extremity trauma.

The topic on preoperative fasting is also of particular importance. Our management is based on the assumption that trauma children are never considered as 'fasting'. Thus, postponing an emergency procedure to wait until the stomach is empty is unnecessary and dangerous and extends the pain of our young patients. Nevertheless, independent of the time interval from the last food intake to trauma and the anaesthesia procedure, equipment and staff for advanced airway management must be available.

The following particularly important implications are associated with the management of minor trauma in children:

- Two anaesthesiologists with particular knowledge in paediatric anaesthesia are required for this kind of treatment.

- Anaesthesiologist A for the block.
- Anaesthesiologist B for the procedural sedation and possible advanced airway management.
- Children are not suitable for novices in ultrasound-guided regional anaesthesia.
- An open communication with the parents and (if possible) with the children provides a trustful basis.
- A preoperative fasting period is not meaningful.
- All ultrasound-guided regional anaesthetic techniques which are described in adults can also be performed in children.
- The sedation can be performed as described in the internal guidelines of the individual medical institution.
- Spontaneous ventilation should always be maintained.
- Careful assisted face mask ventilation does not increase the risk of pulmonary aspiration.
- Equipment for advanced airway management should always be available.

Suggested further reading

Rubin, K., Sullivan, D., Sadhasivam, S., 2009. Are peripheral and neuraxial blocks with ultrasound guidance more effective and safe in children? *Pediatric Anesthesia*, 19(2), pp.92–6.

Chapter 8

Ultrasound appearance of nerves and other anatomical or non-anatomical structures

Adequate interpretation of all anatomical structures in ultrasound is a prerequisite for the correct performance of regional techniques.

8.1 Appearance of nerves in ultrasonography

Recall that 'every nerve has a particular visualization in ultrasonography'. This statement is perhaps more confusing than helpful to the beginner, but ultrasonography is an important method for the safe identification of particular nerves for the experienced user.

On analyzing a histological illustration of a peripheral nerve, the epineurium, perineurium, connective tissue, and neurons are visible. By using high-frequency ultrasound, the visualization of all these structures is possible (Figure 8.1).

Due to the large percentage of neuronal structures, nerve structures appear hypoechoic with a hyperechoic surrounding when visualized in a proximal position (Figure 8.2). The more peripheral the visualized nerve structures, the more hyperechoic the image (Figure 8.3), which can be explained by the increased percentage of connective tissue between neurons.

For the purposes of regional anaesthesia, nerves should always be visualized in a transverse view, appearing as described above. In principle, it is also possible to visualize nerves in a longitudinal view, wherein the internal echotexture is described as a reticular pattern in which longitudinal discontinuous bands are visible (Figure 8.4). However, in daily clinical practice, the longitudinal view is of minor importance.

It is an interesting phenomenon that nerves appear in different forms depending on their anatomical position. One example is the ulnar nerve in the distal upper arm position, and at the proximal and middle forearm (Figure 8.5). Some nerves have a consistent typical form, including the musculocutaneous and radial nerves (depending on the scanning level), but, in principle, all

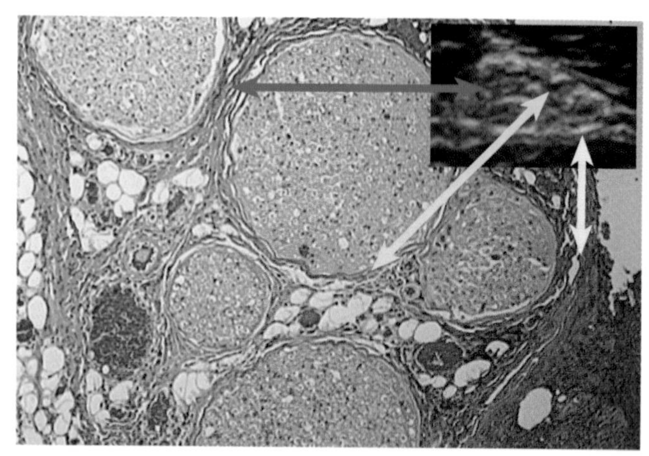

Fig. 8.1 Histological and corresponding ultrasound illustration of a peripheral nerve. White arrow: epineurium; blue arrow: perineurium; yellow arrow: endoneurium.

peripheral nerves appear in individual and typical forms. These forms can be described as round (Figure 8.6), oval (Figure 8.7), or triangular (Figure 8.8). Therefore, the correct description of the ultrasound appearance of peripheral nerves is based on both the echogenicity and form (e.g. hyperechoic and round).

The angle of the probe relative to the nerves is also important. The echogenicity of structures varies according to the angle of the ultrasound beam, a phenomenon known as *anisotropy*. The anisotropic behaviour of peripheral nerves is individual, with the sciatic nerve showing the highest level of variation (Figure 8.9).

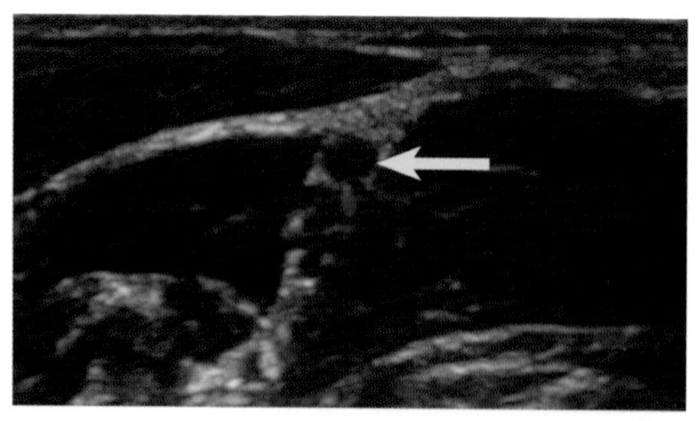

Fig. 8.2 The arrow indicates a hypoechoic central nerve structure (C5 root in the interscalene space) with a hyperechoic border in the area of the interscalene groove. Tracking of this nerve structure in a proximal and distal direction is possible and is an important method of identification.

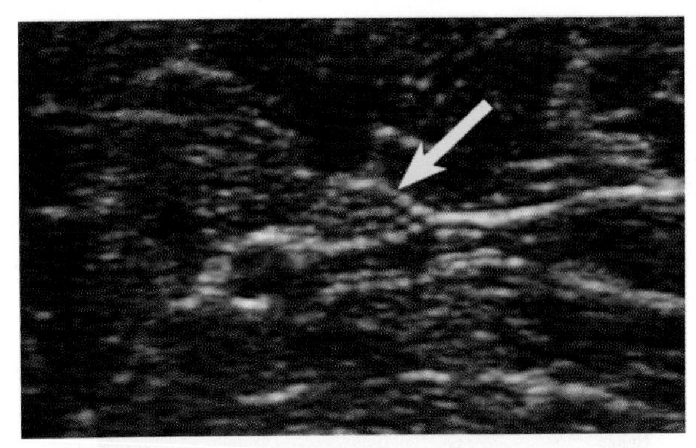

Fig. 8.3 The arrow indicates a hyperechoic peripheral nerve structure (ulnar nerve at the level of the lower third of the forearm). Tracking of this nerve structure in a proximal and distal direction is possible and is an important method of identification.

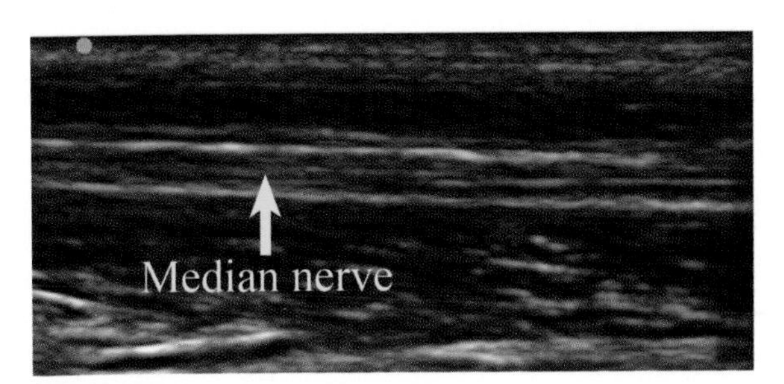

Fig. 8.4 Longitudinal view of a peripheral nerve.

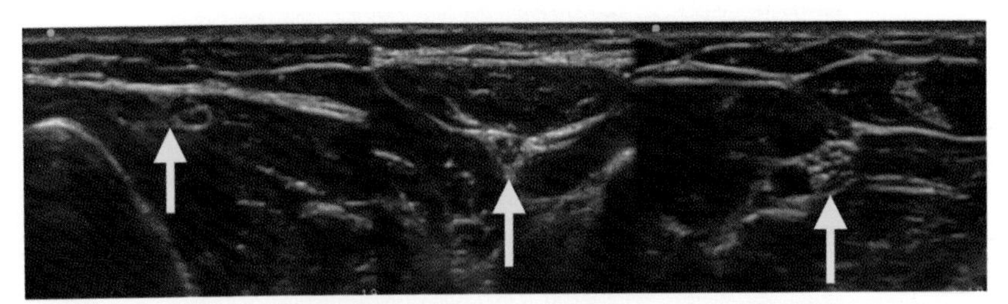

Fig. 8.5 Typical form of the ulnar nerve at three different anatomical positions. Above the elbow joint: oval; proximal third of the forearm: triangular; distal third of the forearm: round.

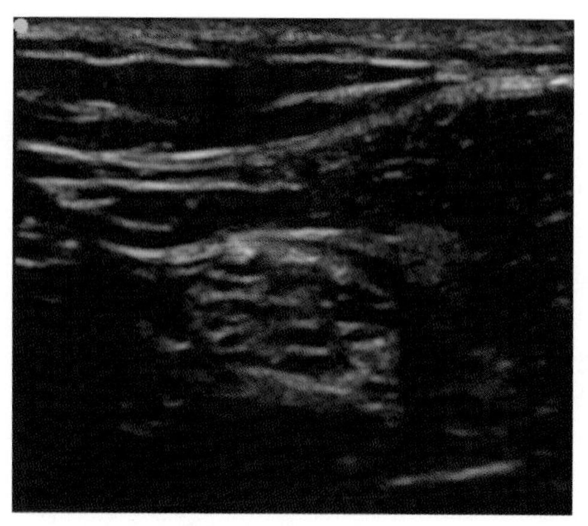

Fig. 8.6 Round shape of a peripheral nerve (tibial nerve at the popliteal level).

8.2 Strategies when nerves are not visible

For certain regional anaesthetic techniques, nerve structures are not (always) directly visible under ultrasound guidance:

- Intercostal.
- Paravertebral.
- Psoas compartment.
- Rectus sheath.
- Transversus abdominis plane (TAP).

The reasons for the impaired or even impossible direct ultrasound visualization of nerve structures with the above techniques are mainly related to the small dimension of nerves, large overlying muscle masses, or overlying bones.

The fact that nerves are not directly visible in some regional techniques is not necessarily associated with more difficulties in practical block performance.

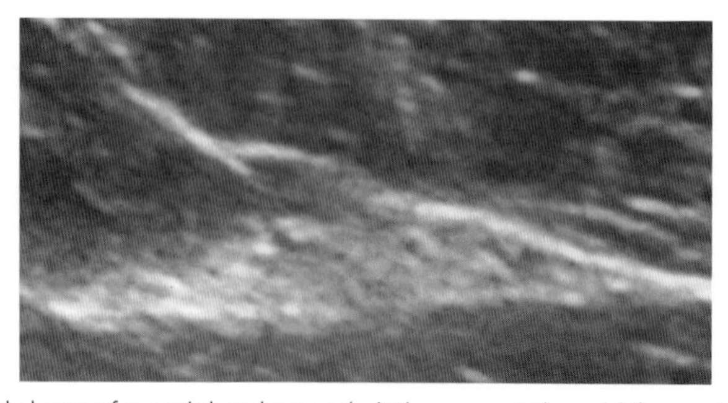

Fig 8.7 Oval shape of a peripheral nerve (sciatic nerve at the mid-femoral level).

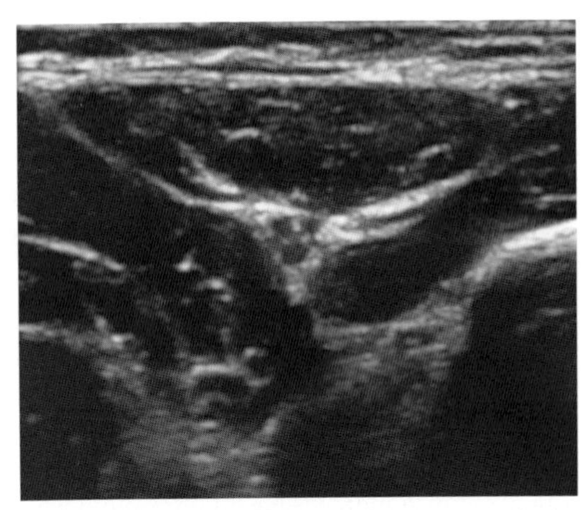

Fig. 8.8 Triangular shape of a peripheral nerve (ulnar nerve at the level of the forearm).

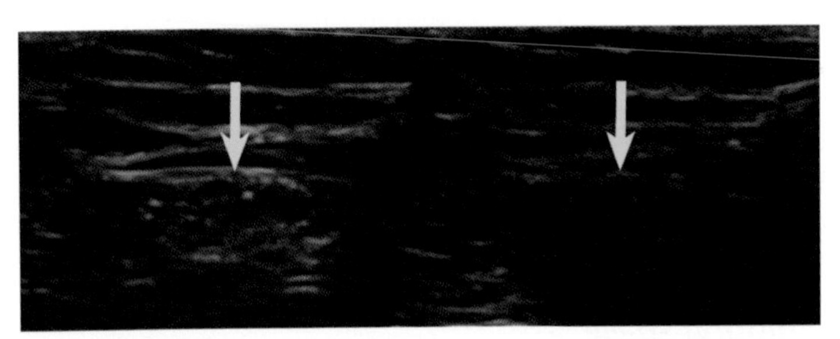

Fig. 8.9 Anisotropic behaviour of a peripheral nerve. On the left side is the sciatic nerve clearly visible; on the right side, the sciatic nerve has disappeared after a 5° movement of the ultrasound probe.

In all techniques above, except the psoas compartment block, the local anaesthetic can be injected between clearly defined muscle layers. The difficulties of the psoas compartment block consist in the depth of the central lumbar plexus, the large overlying muscle masses, and the fact that the nerve structures are not located between muscle layers. The exact techniques of the particular blocks are described in the corresponding chapters.

8.3 Appearance of neuronal-related structures in ultrasonography

8.3.1 Flavum ligament

The flavum ligament inserts inferiorly onto the superior edge and the postero-superior surface of the caudal lamina and superiorly onto the inferior edge and antero-inferior surface of the cephalad lamina. The flavum ligament is composed of a 2.5–3.5mm thick superficial and a 1mm thin deep component. Due to the complexity of this anatomical structure and the extensive contact with osseous structures, it is not surprising that ultrasound visualization is difficult. Figure 8.10 illustrates the flavum ligament in a longitudinal and transverse view in a 1.9kg newborn, compared with the identification via ultrasound in adults which is always impaired (Figure 8.11) and, in some cases, impossible.

8.3.2 Dura mater

The dura mater is the outer part of the meninges and is composed of dense fibrous tissue. It is not connected to osseous structures in the area of the spinal cord and therefore, it is much more visible on ultrasound where it appears as echogenic line in longitudinal views. Depending on the status of ossification, the best ultrasound visibility can be obtained in babies (Figure 8.12) whereas the visibility in adults is impaired (Figure 8.13).

8.3.3 Spinal cord

The spinal cord appears as a grey structure with an internal, longitudinal, streaky pattern (Figure 8.14). Again, depending on the status of ossification, more or less details such as the central canal and the conus (Figure 8.15) are visible in children.

8.3.4 Epidural space

The epidural space is formed between the periost (outer layer of the dura mater), flavum ligament, and dura mater, and contains connective tissue, fat, nerve structures, and vessels (arteries and veins). The ultrasound appearance of the epidural space is more or less isoechoic or slightly hyperechoic relative

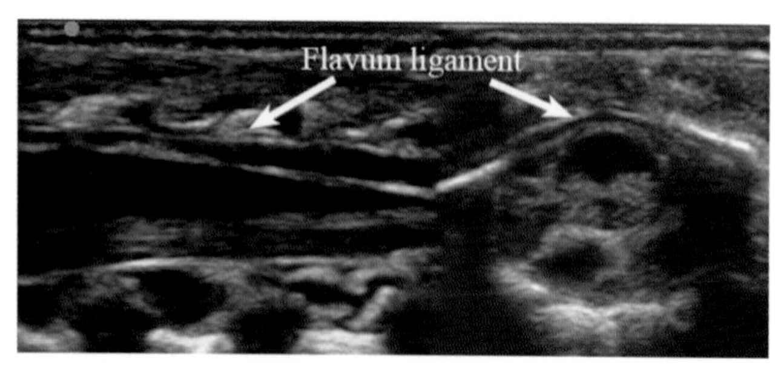

Fig. 8.10 Longitudinal (left) and transverse (right) ultrasound illustration of the flavum ligament in a 1.9kg newborn.

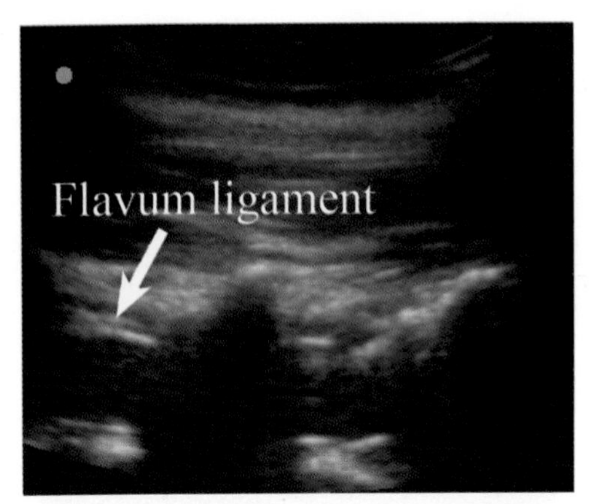

Fig. 8.11 Longitudinal view of the flavum ligament in an adult.

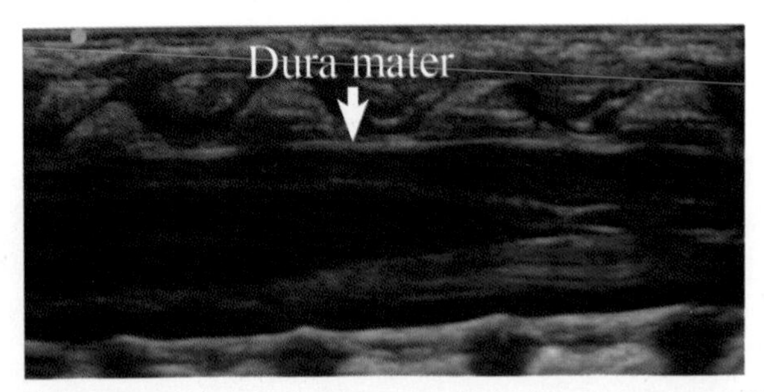

Fig. 8.12 Longitudinal view of the lumbar part of the dura mater in a 1.9kg newborn.

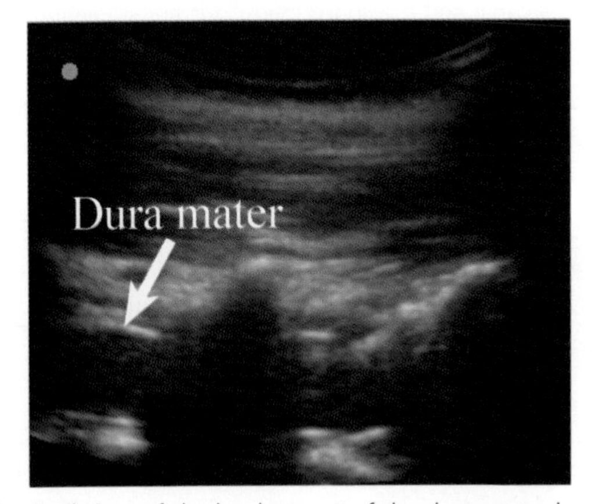

Fig. 8.13 Longitudinal view of the lumbar part of the dura mater in an adult.

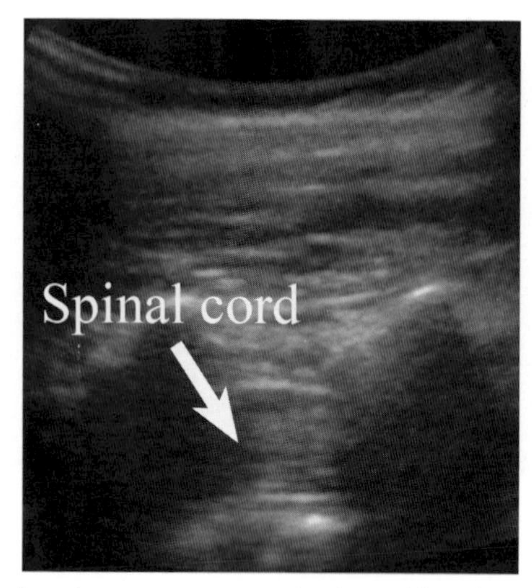

Fig. 8.14 The spinal cord appears as a grey structure with an internal longitudinal streaky pattern.

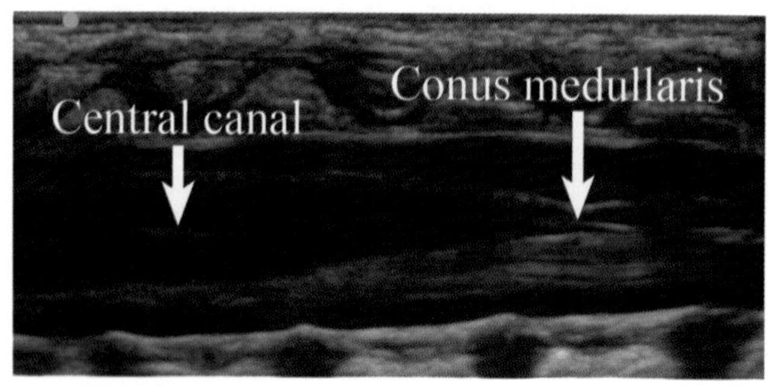

Fig. 8.15 The central canal and the conus medullaris are visible in babies.

to the dorsal structures (flavum ligament, interspinal ligaments). This isoechoic to slightly hyperechoic behaviour (Figure 8.16) is the main reason why the ultrasound technique of epidural puncture should always be performed as a combination between ultrasound guidance and the traditional loss-of-resistance method. Once fluid is administered inside the epidural space, the isoechoic behaviour of this space changes into a more hypoechoic behaviour and the dura mater moves anteriorly (Figure 8.17).

8.3.5 Internal intercostal membrane

The internal intercostal membrane (IIM) is the lateral continuation of the superior costotransverse ligament, is a strong fibrous band and is the posterior

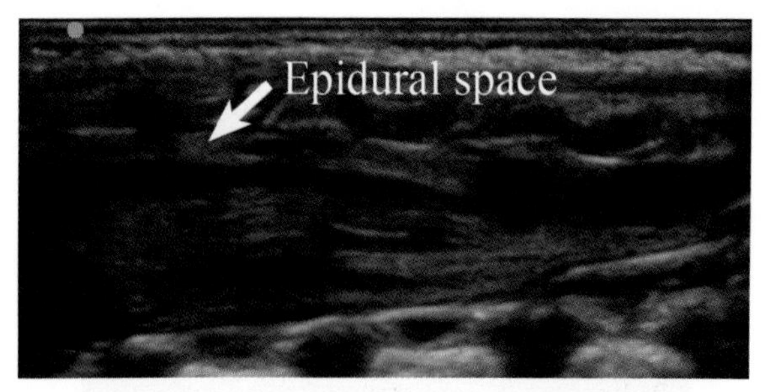

Fig. 8.16 Slightly hyperechoic ultrasound behaviour of the epidural space.

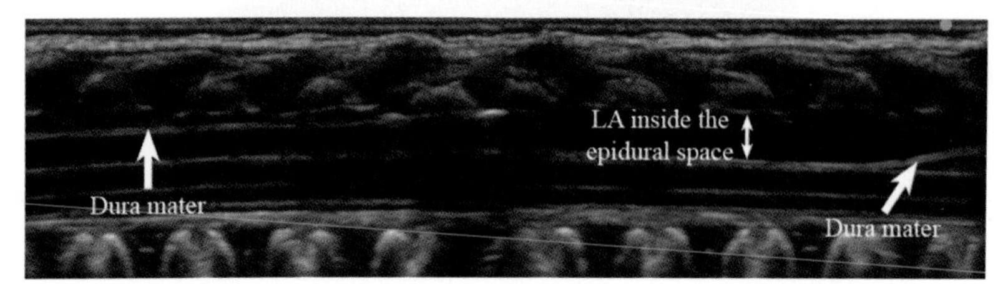

Fig. 8.17 Downward movement of the dura mater in a 3kg newborn during administration of local anaesthetic (LA) (appears hypoechoic between the flavum ligament and the dura mater). Left: before administration of LA; right: during administration of LA.

boundary of the paravertebral space. It arises from the neck of a rib to the transverse process of the vertebra above. The ultrasound appearance of the IIM is a double layer-like structure (Figure 8.18).

8.4 Appearance of other anatomical structures in ultrasound

In addition to correct ultrasound-guided interpretation of neuronal structures, it is also important to correctly recognize adjacent anatomical structures. This particular knowledge is mandatory for the correct performance of blocks and to avoid complications.

8.4.1 Tendons

In the transverse view, the ultrasonographic appearance of tendons is similar to that of nerves (Figure 8.19). An excellent method for a clear discrimination of these structures is to track them over a certain distance; tendons disappear over distances whereas nerves should be visible in their entirety. Using a longitudinal view, the internal structure of tendons is visualized as longitudinal,

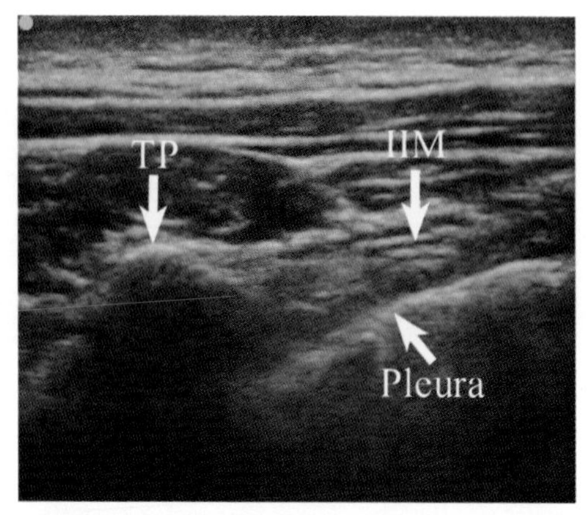

Fig. 8.18 Ultrasound illustration of the paravertebral space between the internal intercostal membrane (IIM), the transverse process (TP), and the pleura.

continuous, hypoechoic bands with hyperechoic, intertendinous septae (fibrillar pattern) (Figure 8.20).

8.4.2 Blood vessels

The safe identification of blood vessels is of particular importance. Discrimination of arteries and veins is possible with colour Doppler imaging (Figure 8.21). An additional and simple method to discriminate arteries from veins is to increase the contact pressure of the probe: veins are compressible, but arteries retain their rounded shape (Figure 8.22). However, a practical

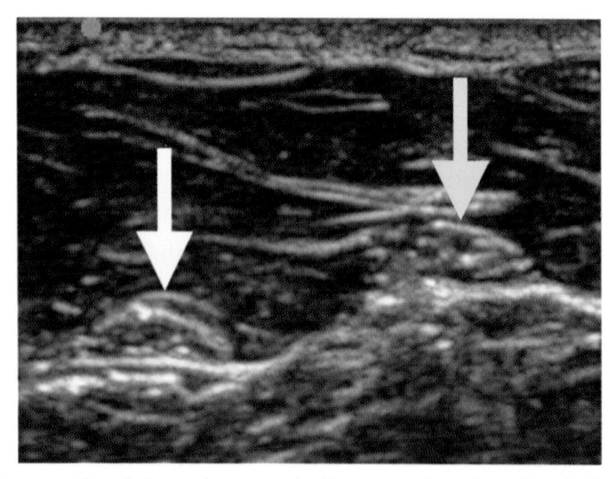

Fig. 8.19 Cross-sectional view of a nerve (yellow arrow) and tendon (white arrow). Discrimination is only possible by tracking the structures in a proximal direction where the tendon disappears.

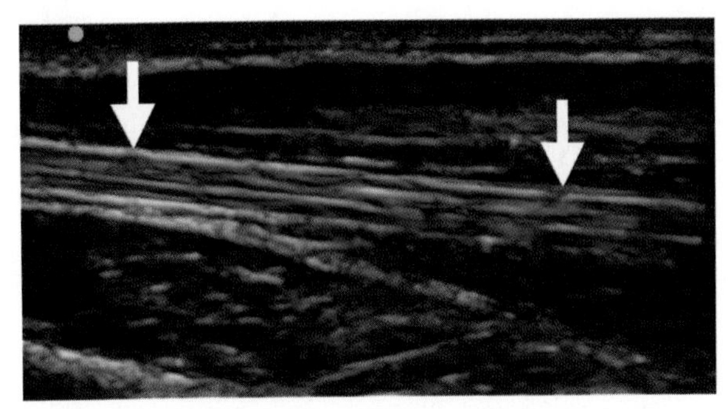

Fig. 8.20 Typical longitudinal view of a tendon.

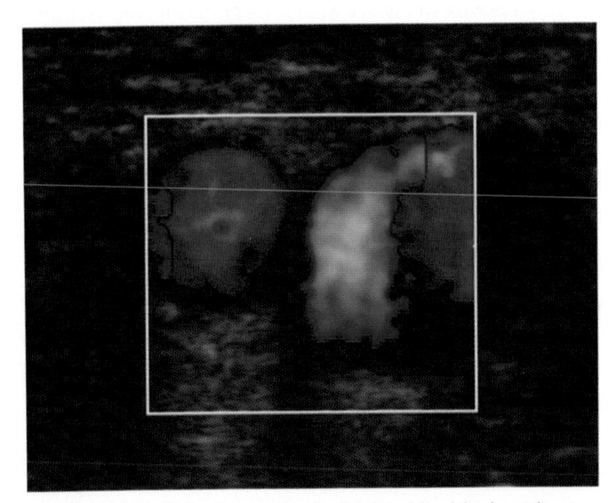

Fig. 8.21 Colour Doppler of the femoral vein (right side: blue) and artery (left side: red).

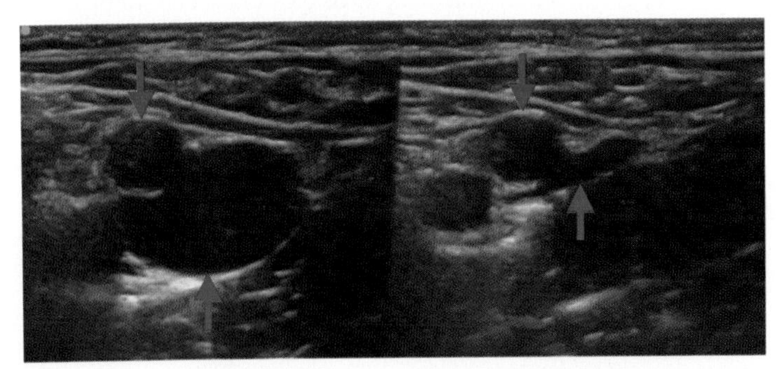

Fig. 8.22 Non-compressed (left) and compressed (right) femoral vessels. Red arrow: artery; blue arrow: vein.

implication of this is that there is a risk of inadvertent and unnoticed puncture of the vein due to high probe-related contact pressure. Direct observation of the spread of local anaesthetic during injection is absolutely mandatory to avoid intravascular drug administration.

Blood vessels can also serve as guidance structures to facilitate the location of nerves. The infraclavicular portions of the brachial plexus or the femoral nerve lateral to the femoral artery are prime examples.

8.4.3 Muscles

Muscles may appear in ultrasound images either as slightly heterogeneous structures with band-like, hyperechoic, intramuscular septae (Figure 8.23) or as homogeneous structures (Figure 8.24). In general, muscles show a fibrolamellar, ultrasonographic appearance. Muscle tissue is often the main reference structure regarding the echogenicity of nerves. It is helpful to assign the different muscle structures relative to the nerves.

8.4.4 Bones

The cortex of bony structures appears as a hyperechoic structure and the contour of the cortex may serve as a guidance structure for specific block techniques (e.g. deep cervical plexus or paravertebral blockade). Due to the fact that the ultrasound beam is totally reflected by the cortex, the areas behind the cortex are completely anechoic (dorsal ultrasound shadow). Figure 8.25 illustrates the appearance of a bony structure in ultrasonography.

8.4.5 Pleura

Pleura (physiologic thickness of 0.1mm) appear as a hyperechoic structure (Figure 8.26) and usually follow the cycle of breathing. Movement of the pleura is minimal at the apex, which is of particular importance during the performance of periclavicular brachial plexus blockade. The subpleural tissues

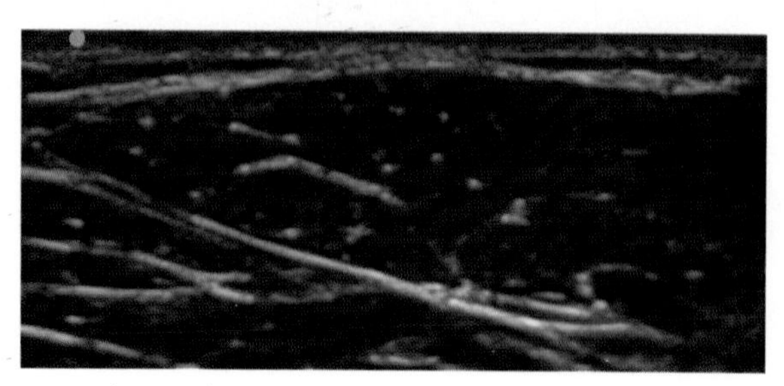

Fig. 8.23 Heterogenic muscle appearance with band-like hyperechoic intramuscular septae.

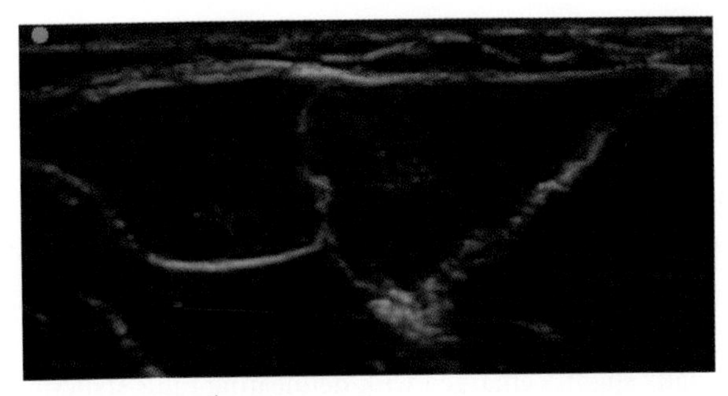

Fig. 8.24 Homogenous muscle appearance.

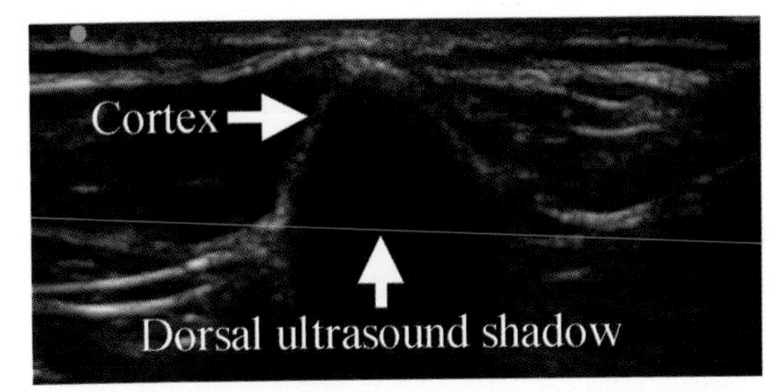

Fig. 8.25 Ultrasonographic appearance of the humerus. The cortex of the bone appears hyperechoic with an anechoic dorsal ultrasound shadow.

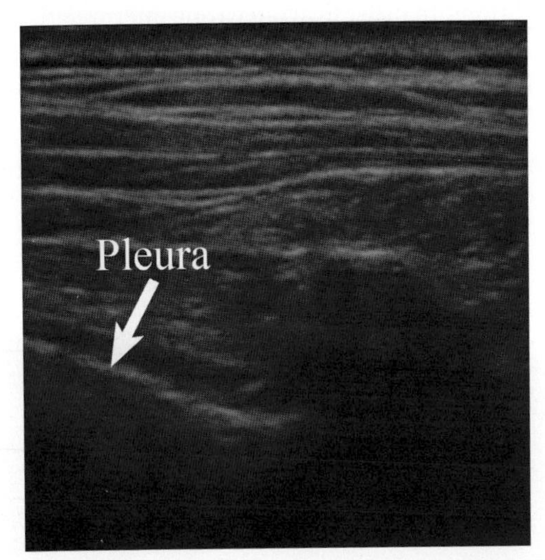

Fig. 8.26 Typical ultrasound appearance of the pleura at the paravertebral thoracic region.

are difficult to delineate and to differentiate, even with high-resolution ultrasound. Pleural effusion, inflammation, various pathologies, and pneumothorax are detectable by ultrasound.

8.4.6 Lymph nodes

Lymph nodes appear oval- or bean-shaped with a hyperechoic, vascularized hilus entering the lymph node from its border (Figure 8.27). Lymph nodes are typically depicted as having a longitudinal diameter of 2–3mm. Reactive lymph nodes are usually slightly enlarged with delineating hilus structures and have an oval appearance. Malignant lymph nodes are usually round, show no hilus structures, and have a low echogenicity.

8.4.7 Local anaesthetic

Local anaesthetic solution appears anechoic in ultrasonography (Figure 8.28). Improved identification of nerve structures is often possible after the administration of local anaesthetic (Figure 8.29).

8.5 Appearance of artefacts in ultrasound

Artefacts refer to physical or technical structures visible in the ultrasound image that have no anatomical correlate. These structures are the result of discrepancies between the ideal tissue used for image calculation and the real object of examination. In general, these artefacts can make the interpretation of images and tissues very difficult; sometimes, however, they can help diagnose certain conditions. In order to avoid wrong interpretation, it is important to examine structures that appear pathological in at least two ultrasound planes. Real structures will be visible in both while artefacts cannot be reproduced.

The most important artefacts are also explained in the section below (also see Section 1.8).

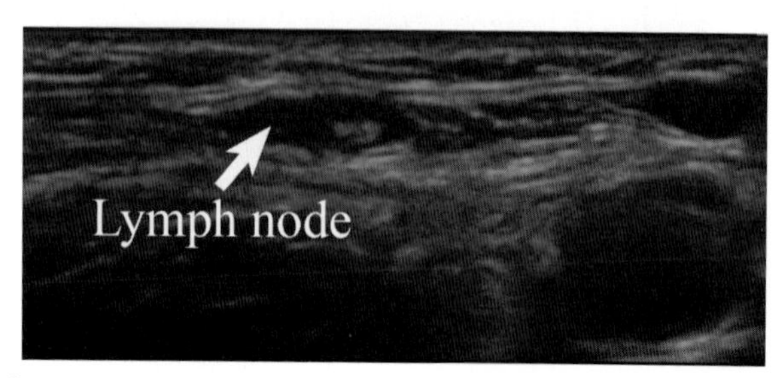

Fig. 8.27 Inflammatory lymph node in the inguinal area.

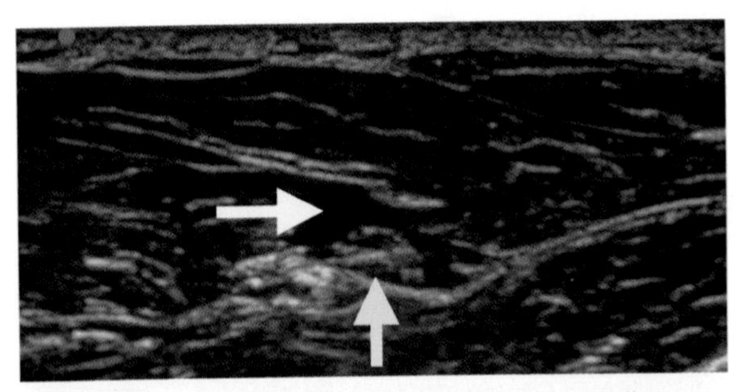

Fig. 8.28 Ultrasonographic visualization of local anaesthetic. Yellow arrow: median nerve; white arrow: hypoechoic appearance of local anaesthetic.

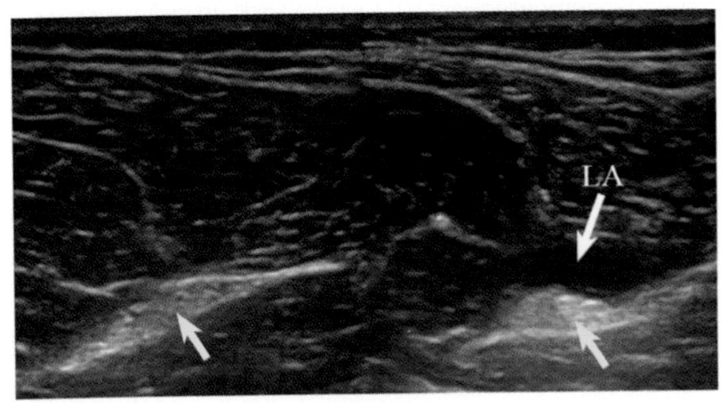

Fig. 8.29 Ultrasonographic appearance of the sciatic nerve before (left) and after (right) administration of LA.

8.5.1 Dorsal enhancement

This is dorsal echo-gaining, e.g. in the dorsal region of a vessel or a cyst (Figure 8.30). It occurs because the content of these structures is mainly liquid and therefore, the attenuation is very low or zero.

8.5.2 Reflection

Reflection occurs if a sound wave meets a border from two different impedances. If the angle of incidence is below 90°, part of the energy will be reflected away from the transducer and the other part will be refracted. If the angle of incidence is perpendicular, part of the energy will be reflected back to the transducer and the other part is been transmitted into deeper regions.

8.5.3 Air

Air has a much lower speed of sound and therefore, total beam reflection occurs on the border between tissue and air. Therefore, no echo information can be detected from the dorsal region (Figure 8.31).

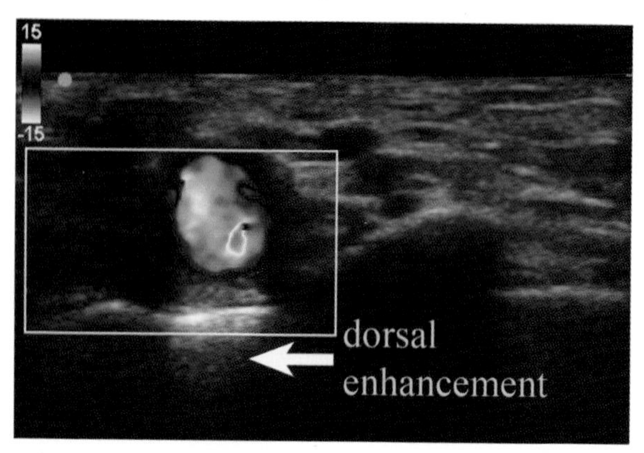

Fig. 8.30 Dorsal enhancement (hyperechoic area) behind the subclavian artery.

8.5.4 Reverberations

Reverberations are artefacts caused when sound waves are multiple-reflected between a reflector in the tissue and the transducer surface (Figure 8.32).

8.5.5 Mirror

Mirroring occurs if a sound wave meets a borderline (significant difference in impedance, e.g. the diaphragm may cause this kind of artefact) and dorsal to this impedance, the same echo information can be detected in the anterior, thus being interpreted as a mirror (Figure 8.33).

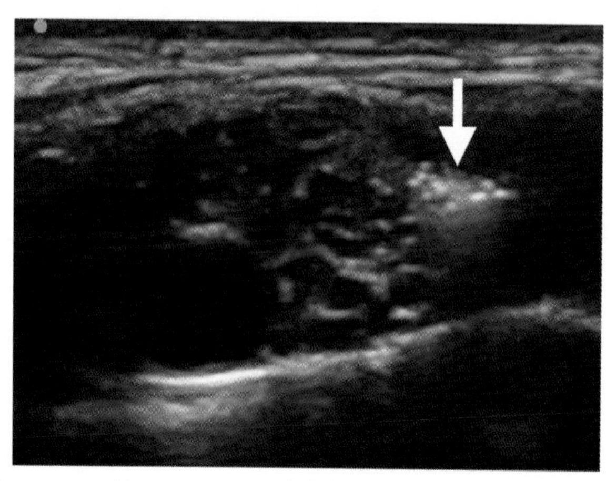

Fig 8.31 Ultrasonographic appearance of air bubbles (white arrow) with dorsal shadow.

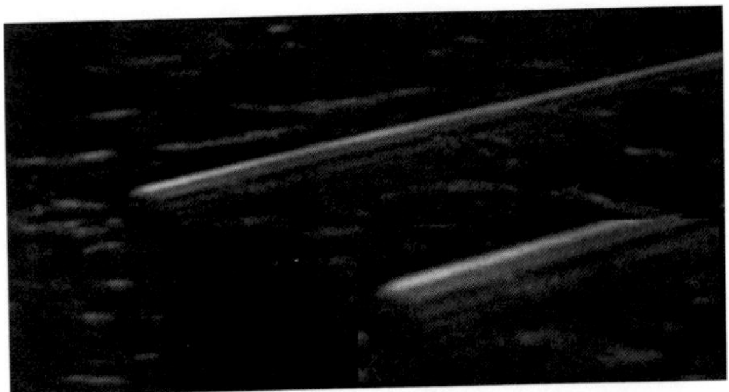

Fig. 8.32 Reverberation artefact caused during an IP needle guidance technique. The artefacts behind the needle are enlarged in the left lower corner.

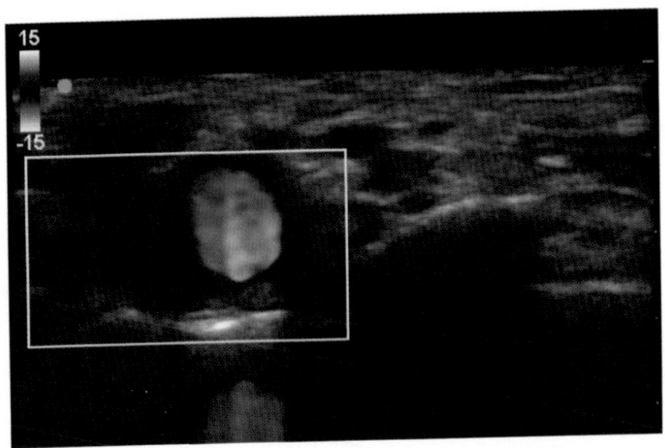

Fig. 8.33 Mirror artefact of the subclavian artery in the area of the supraclavicular brachial plexus.

Suggested further reading

Sites, B., Brull, R., Chan, V., Spence, B., Gallagher, J., Beach, M., Sites, V., Abbas, S., Hartmann, G., 2007. Artefacts and pitfall errors associated with ultrasound-guided regional anaesthesia. Part II: a pictorial approach to understanding and avoidance. *Regional Anesthesia and Pain Medicine*, 32(5), 419–33.

Chapter 9

Needle guidance techniques

The practicability of ultrasound-guided regional blocks has always been equated to the visualization of the needle. Despite the fact that the neuronal structures are blocked by the local anaesthetic and not by the tip of the needle, adequate visualization of needles is mandatory for safe and effective blocks. In addition, the observation of the spread of local anaesthetic is equally important for the performance of regional blocks.

In fact, direct needle visibility is only one aspect of the safety of block performance. From the first descriptions of ultrasonographic-guided regional techniques, most of the authors, in particular those from the Anglo-American areas, favoured the in-plane (IP) techniques where the entire needle should be visualized longitudinal to the scanning head. A good example for such a technical controversy is the interscalene brachial plexus approach from posterior (the so-called 'Pippa approach'). It is important to know that two nerves run inside the median scalene muscle: the longer thoracic and dorsal scapulae nerves. Both nerves can be damaged on piercing the middle scalene muscle when an IP technique is used for interscalene brachial plexus blockade with the possible consequence of a paralysis of the serratus anterior muscle. The out-of-plane (OOP) technique, where the needle is advanced along the course of the posterior interscalene groove, is much more consequent from an anatomical point of view. On the other hand, an IP needle guidance technique should be performed for the supraclavicular approach to the brachial plexus, mainly for technical (it is difficult to obtain the correct angle with the cannula from the medial side where the neck is located) and safety (cervical pleura!) reasons.

It does not really matter for a lot of approaches if an OOP or IP needle guidance technique is used. Peripheral nerve blocks can be performed in a safe and effective way with both techniques. But some particular techniques (see above) are simply more reasonable from anatomical and safety points of view. Detractors may argue that these considerations are not supported by the literature, but daily clinical practice confirms the practicability of particular needle guidance techniques for selective blocks.

As we have seen, there are two different needle guidance techniques used for ultrasound-guided nerve blocks: OOP and IP. These techniques describe the position of the needle relative to the ultrasound probe. In principle, both techniques can be used for most blocks, but anatomical implications require that each specific block technique should be preferentially performed with IP or OOP.

9.1 Out-of-plane (OOP) needle guidance technique

In the OOP technique, the needle is positioned along the short axis of the ultrasound probe (Figure 9.1). Depending on the depth of the target structure, the angle of the needle has to be adjusted. A flat angle is suitable for superficial target structures whereas deep target structures require steeper angles. Only the tip of the needle can be visualized by using the OOP technique (Figure 9.2). Steeper angles are associated with a better visibility of the tip of the needle and compared with flat angles (Figure 9.3).

9.2 In-plane (IP) needle guidance technique

In the IP technique, the needle is positioned along the long axis of the ultrasound probe (Figure 9.4). Historically, most peripheral blocks were performed using the IP technique, but in recent years, the blocks have been adapted to meet anatomical requirements. The IP technique necessitates that the needle is located inside a 1mm longitudinal area. Only slight deviations in a lateral direction can cause the needle to disappear from the ultrasound window.

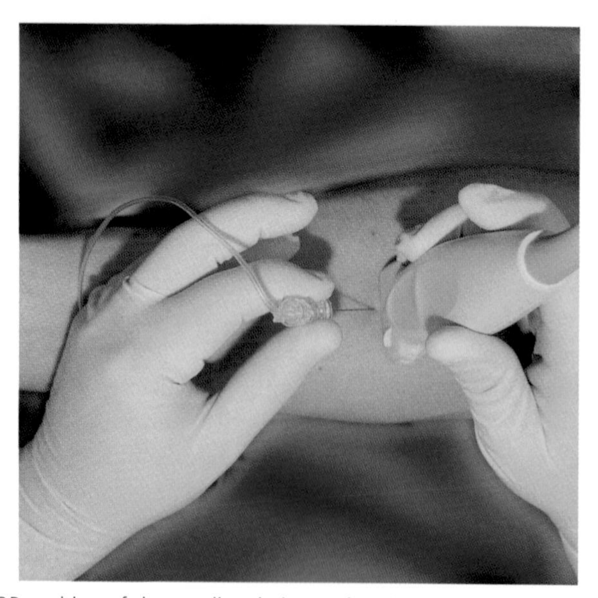

Fig. 9.1 OOP position of the needle relative to the ultrasound probe.

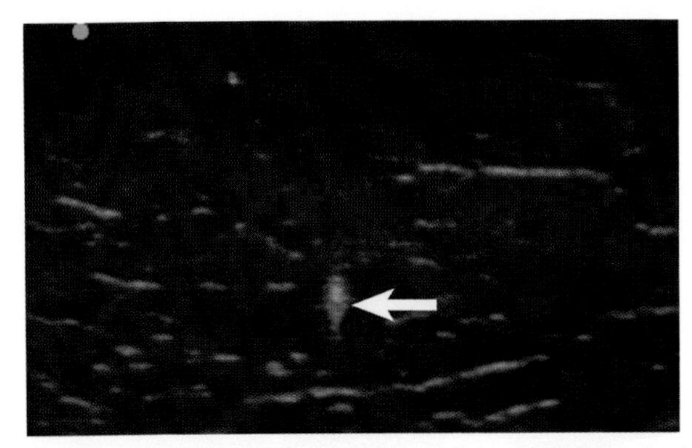

Fig. 9.2 Ultrasonographic appearance of the tip of the needle (arrow) when the OOP technique is used.

Thus, the IP technique needs excellent hand-eye coordination on the part of the physician.

Tools for facilitating the appearance of needles during the IP technique are available, but are associated with the drawback of impaired needle flexibility. The maximal degree of reverberation artefacts is also observed when these kinds of needle guidance tools are used.

It is important to notice that the ultrasound appearance of the needle is significantly better when the angle of insertion is flat compared with a steep angle (Figure 9.5). Recent advancements in needle technology facilitate the ultrasound visibility for steep angles as well (Figure 9.6).

Advancing the needle using the IP technique produces reverberation artefacts and impairs the detection of structures below the body of the needle. These artefacts can be avoided by slight lateral movement of the needle (Figure 9.7).

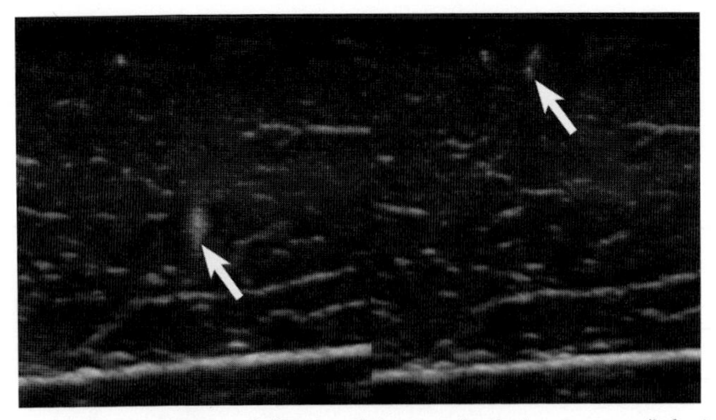

Fig. 9.3 Improved appearance of the tip of the needle during a steep (left side) compared with a flat (right side) angle when the OOP technique is performed.

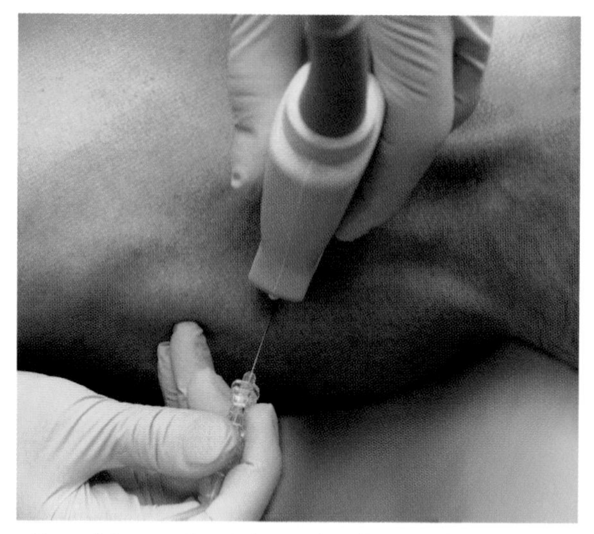

Fig. 9.4 IP position of the needle relative to the ultrasound probe.

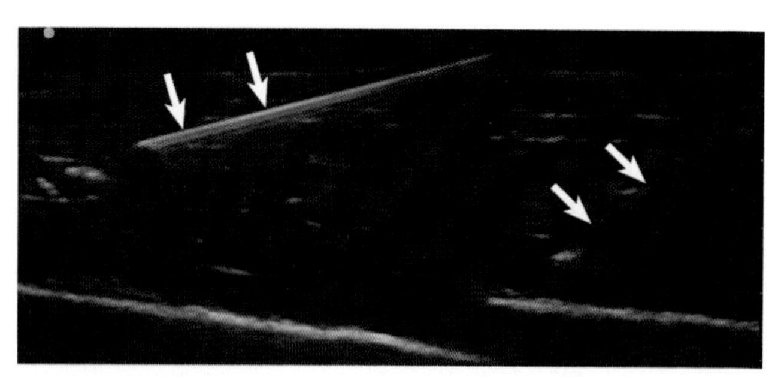

Fig. 9.5 Improved visibility of the body of the needle during a flat (left side) vs a steep (right side) angle when the IP technique is performed.

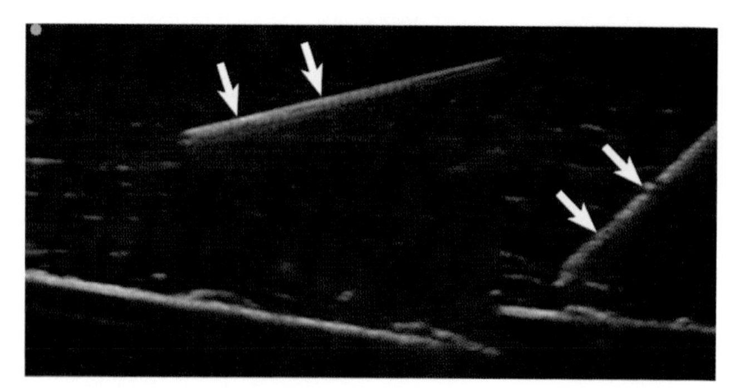

Fig. 9.6 Recent evolutions in needle design allow better visibility for steep angles during the IP needle guidance technique.

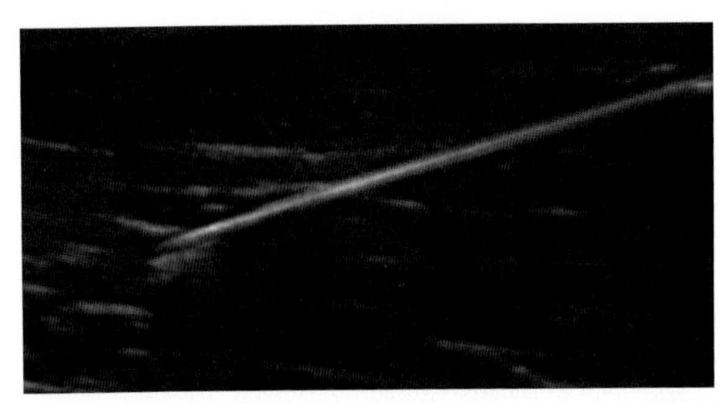

Fig. 9.7 Reverberation artefacts during the IP technique can be avoided by slight lateral movement of the needle relative to the probe.

In addition, the insertion-to-target distance is two- to three-fold longer compared with the OOP technique. Nevertheless, we have defined specific indications for the IP technique (e.g. supraclavicular approach to the brachial plexus, popliteal approach to the sciatic nerve, etc.).

9.3 How to approach a nerve?

Nerve blocks should be performed with the tip of the needle as close to the epineurium as possible. In other words, an *extra-epineural needle tip position* is, from today's point of view, safe and effective. Usually, some connective tissue lies between the place where the local anaesthetic is administered and

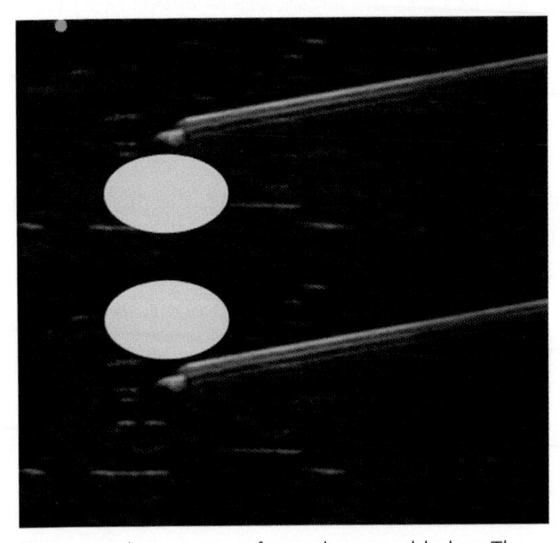

Fig. 9.8 Correct IP approach to a nerve from above and below.The nerves are simulated by yellow ovals.

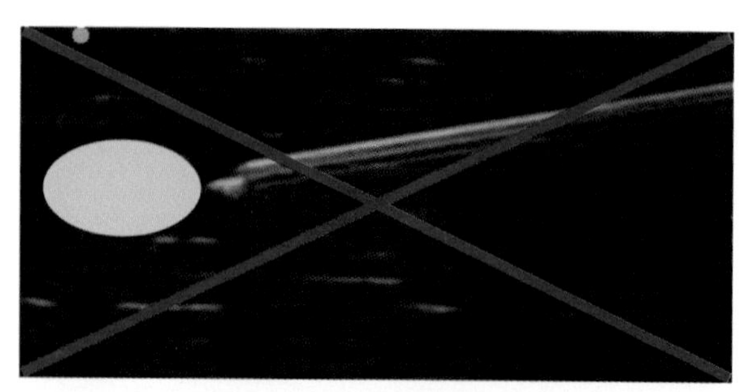

Fig. 9.9 Direct approach to a nerve should be avoided. The nerve is simulated by a yellow oval.

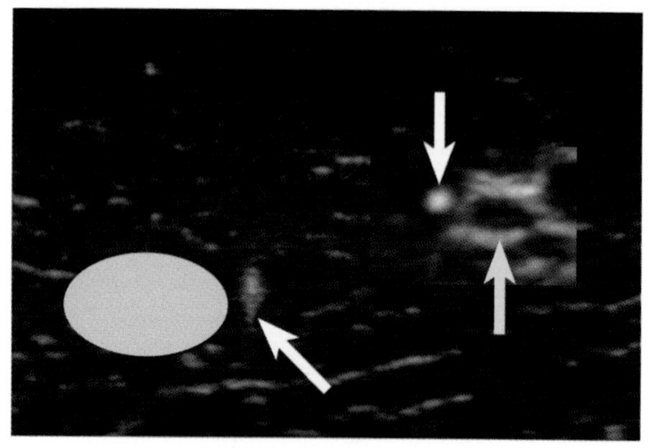

Fig. 9.10 Two examples of a correct lateral approach to nerves during the OOP technique. White arrows: tip of the needle; yellow arrow: hypoechoic C5 root; yellow oval: simulation of a nerve.

the epineurium. Whether the amount of connective tissue influences the qualities of blocks remains unclear.

By using the IP needle guidance technique, the nerve structures should be approached from above or below (Figure 9.8), whereas a direct approach should be avoided due to an inadvertent intra-epineural needle tip position (Figure 9.9). Figure 9.10 illustrates the correct position of the needle tip during the OOP needle guidance technique.

Chapter 10

Pearls and pitfalls

10.1 Setting and orientation of the probe

The position of the anaesthesiologist relative to the patient should be 'face-to-face' with the ultrasound machine positioned lateral to the head of the patient (Figure 10.1). For approaches at the neck, the anaesthesiologist might wish to position themselves behind the head of the patient (Figure 10.2). The orientation of the probe should adhere to a 'true image' (i.e. the left side of the probe equates to the left side of the screen).

10.2 Pressure during injection

High-pressure injection of local anaesthetic is associated with neuronal damage and should always be avoided. During the performance of specific blocks, e.g. in the axillary approach to the brachial plexus where anatomical structures are in close proximity to each other, high-pressure injection can eventually be detected. Where high-pressure injection is detected, the pressure can be alleviated by minimal withdrawal of the needle.

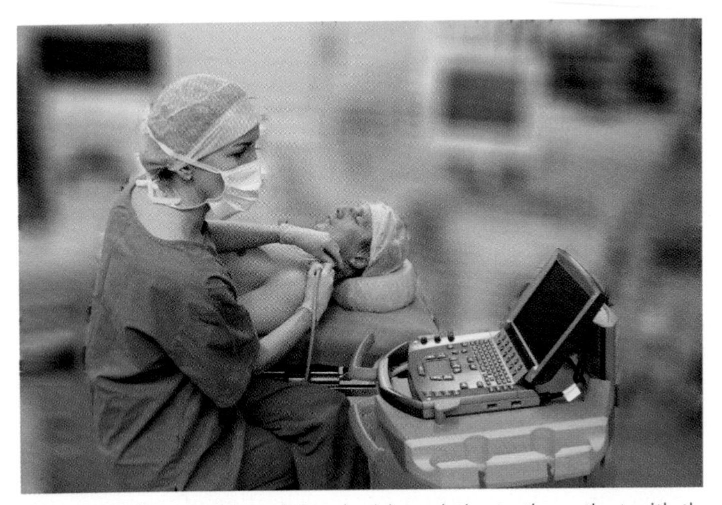

Fig. 10.1 'Face-to-face' position of the physician relative to the patient with the ultrasound machine lateral to the head of the patient.

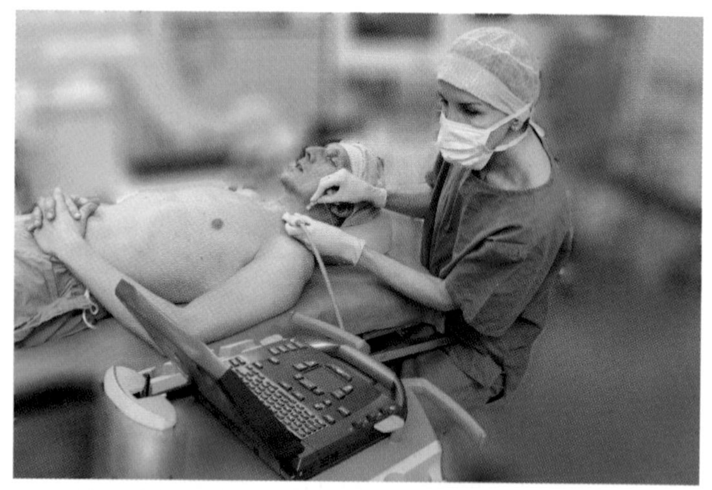

Fig. 10.2 Position of the physician behind the patient.

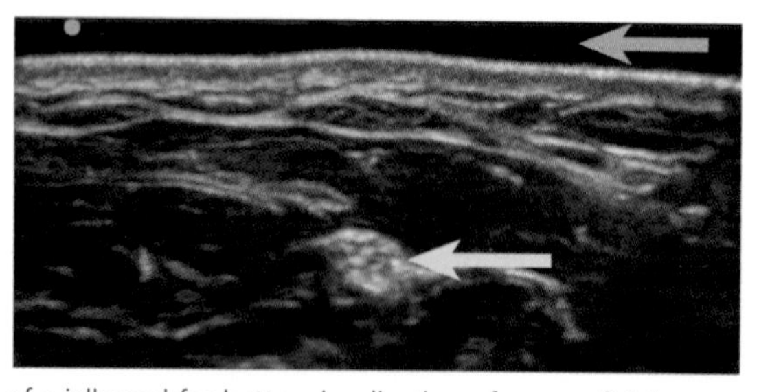

Fig. 10.3 Use of a jelly pad for better visualization of a superficial anatomical structure. Yellow arrow: median nerve; grey arrow: anechoic area due to the 0.5mm jelly pad.

Equipment for the detection of pressure during injection is available, but is not introduced in daily clinical practice due to the lack of a specific measured value where an intraneuronal injection can be safely detected.

10.3 Jelly pad for extreme superficial structures

For an improved ultrasonographic visualization of very superficial structures (e.g. superficial branch of the peroneus nerve), a sterile jelly pad may be used to increase the distance from the probe to the skin. A jelly pad also has the advantage that it is totally free of artefacts caused by the traditional application of jelly. This can be important when scanning tiny nerves as even the smallest artefacts may prevent the appropriate visualization of the target structures (Figure 10.3).

Chapter 11

Nerve supply of big joints

Most surgical procedures managed with regional anaesthesia are performed at or around big joints. Thus, it was the authors' intention to provide fundamental information concerning the nerve supply of the big joints (shoulder, elbow, wrist, hip, knee, and ankle). This chapter should support clinical decisions for surgical anaesthesia or pain therapy. Nevertheless, this chapter cannot replace anatomical textbooks in that particular field.

11.1 Shoulder joint

The shoulder joint is mainly innervated by small articular branches derived from the muscular branches to the muscles adhering and tensioning the joint capsule. The suprascapular nerve gives off articular branches to the anterior aspect whereas the proximal and posterior parts of the joint receive fibres from the muscular branches to the supraspinatus, infraspinatus, and teres minor muscles via the suprascapular nerve. Recurrent fibres from the infraclavicular brachial plexus supply the inferior aspect of the joint near the humerus. These fibres are from the musculocutaneous nerve anteriorly and the axillary nerve posteriorly and at the axillary recessus, and occasionally from the posterior fascicle. Sympathetic fibres originate mainly from the stellate ganglion and the perivascular sympathetic network surrounding the subclavian and axillary arteries.

11.1.1 Major nerve supply of the shoulder joint

- Suprascapular nerve
- Musculocutaneous nerve
- Axillary nerve.

11.2 Elbow joint

Articular branches of all four main nerves of the upper extremity supply the joint capsule of the elbow joint. The median, musculocutaneous, and radial nerves innervate the anterior part of the elbow joint via direct articular branches (median nerve) and small fibres originating from muscular branches (radial nerve, musculocutaneous nerve). The dorsal area of the joint is innervated in the same manner by fibres from the ulnar and radial nerves.

11.2.1 Major nerve supply of the elbow joint

- Median nerve.
- Musculocutaneous nerve.
- Radial nerve.
- Ulnar nerve.

11.3 Wrist

Sensory innervation of the wrist is established by the adjacent nerves. Additionally, numerous connections exist between the small articular branches of their respective nerves. The palmar region receives articular branches of the ulnar, median, and anterior interosseous nerves (median nerve). The radial aspect of the wrist is innervated by the dorsal lateral antebrachial cutaneous branch and the superficial branch (both from the radial nerve). The latter nerves extend to the dorsum of the wrist which is mainly supplied by the dorsal interosseous nerve (radial nerve). The dorsal ramus of the ulnar nerve gives off branches to ulnar side of the wrist.

11.3.1 Major nerve supply of wrist

- Ulnar nerve.
- Median nerve.
- Radial nerve.

11.4 Hip joint

Both the lumbar and sacral plexus are involved in the innervation of the hip joint. The femoral and obturator nerves supply the anterior aspect whereas the sacral plexus innervates the posterior aspect of the hip joint.

11.4.1 Major nerve supply of the hip joint

- Femoral nerve.
- Obturator nerve.
- Sciatic nerve.

11.5 **Knee joint**

The joint capsule of the knee is innervated by articular branches of all adjacent nerves, including the obturator nerve. The anteromedial region is innervated by fibres from a muscular branch to the vastus medialis muscle (femoral nerve), and by the obturator, saphenous, and tibial nerves. The anterolateral region receives fibres from a muscular branch to the vastus lateralis muscle (femoral nerve), and the tibial and peroneal nerves (recurrent branches). The posterior branch of the obturator nerve as well as the tibial nerve and recurrent branches of the common peroneal nerve supply the dorsal region of the knee joint. Articular branches of the obturator nerve may arise from the anterior or posterior branch. They form a plexus around the popliteal artery and pass distally with a branch of the latter reaching the joint capsule.

11.5.1 **Major nerve supply of the knee joint**

- Obturator nerve.
- Femoral nerve.
- Saphenous nerve.
- Tibial nerve.
- Peroneal nerve.

11.6 **Ankle**

The saphenous, tibial, and deep peroneal nerves give off articular branches to the medial side of the ankle. Articular branches of the sural and deep peroneal nerves innervate the lateral side of the ankle.

11.6.1 **Major nerve supply of the ankle**

- Saphenous nerve.
- Tibial nerve.
- Deep peroneal nerve.
- Sural nerve.

Chapter 12

Neck blocks

12.1 General anatomical considerations

The cervical plexus is formed by the ventral rami of the spinal nerves C1–4. In this context, only the rami of nerves C2–4 are of interest for regional anaesthetic purposes. Each nerve (except the first) divides into an ascending and descending branch to form three communicating loops. The cervical plexus is located at the level of the first four cervical vertebrae, deep beneath the internal jugular vein and anterior to the levator scapulae and middle scalene muscles. The cervical plexus is covered by the sternocleidomastoideus muscle. The branches of the cervical plexus can be classified as either deep or superficial (Figure 12.1).

12.2 Deep cervical plexus blockade

12.2.1 Anatomy

The deep branches of the cervical plexus can be further subdivided into internal and external series. The internal series is formed by communicating branches consisting of several filaments which pass from the loops between the upper cervical nerves to the vagus and hypoglossus nerves and the sympathetic trunk. Muscular branches supply the longus capitis, rectus capitis lateralis, and anterior muscles. Cervical communicant filaments from the second and third cervical nerves pass downwards to the lateral side of the internal jugular vein, crossing in front of it at the middle of the neck to form a loop with the descending ramus of the hypoglossus nerve (ansa hypoglossi). Another component of the internal series is the phrenic nerve which mainly arises from the ventral ramus of nerve C4. It passes obliquely on the ventral surface of the anterior scalene muscle, beneath the sternocleidomastoideus and omohyoideus muscles. Finally, it passes between the subclavian vessels and subsequently enters the thorax.

The external series of the deep cervical plexus communicates with the accessory nerve. Muscular branches are distributed to the sternocleidomastoideus, trapezius, levator scapulae, and median scalene muscles.

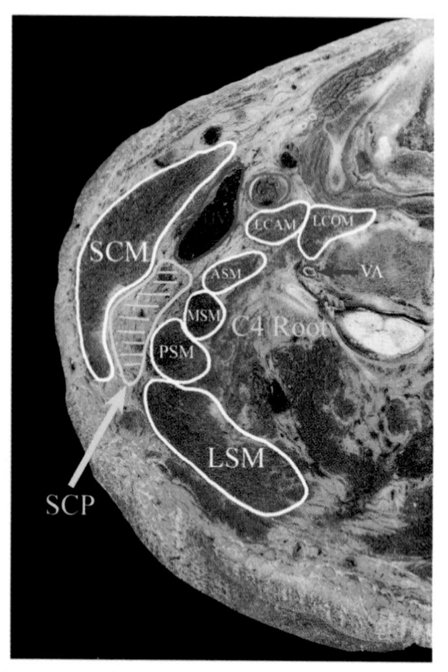

Fig. 12.1 Anatomical cross-sectional view of the neck with the C4 root (between the anterior and posterior tubercles of the C4 transverse process) representing one part of the deep cervical plexus and with the superficial cervical plexus behind the sternocleidomastoid muscle. SCP: superficial cervical plexus; SCM: sternocleidomastoid muscle; LSM: levator scapulae muscle; PSM: posterior scalene muscle; MSM: middle scalene muscle; ASM: anterior scalene muscle; LCAM: longus capitis muscle; LCOM: longus colli muscle; CA: carotic artery; IJV: internal jugular vein; VA: vertebral artery; left side=lateral.

12.2.2 **Anatomical variations**

The anatomical position of the vertebral artery at the level of the upper cervical vertebrae is highly variable. Regardless of this, however, the vertebral artery is in close proximity to the nerve structures. The location of the ansa hypoglossi also varies. It is usually situated between the sternocleidomastoideus muscle and the carotid artery superficial to the internal jugular vein, but it may also be located between the carotid artery and the internal jugular or, in rare cases, dorsal to both vessels. The ansa hypoglossi also varies in length; it may end below the level of the thyroid or at the level of the hyoid bone.

12.2.3 **Ultrasound guidance technique**

The position of the probe is strictly lateral at the level of the brachial plexus. Once the C5 root is detected and tracked backwards from an area of the posterior interscalene groove to the transverse process, the probe should be advanced cranially until the C4 root appears (Figure 12.2). Both the anterior and posterior tuberculi have a characteristic contour on ultrasonography. The early division of the anterior ramus of the C4 root into a cervical and brachial branch can usually be detected (Figure 12.3), and similarly for the phrenic nerve. The roots of nerves C2 and C3 can be visualized in an analogue procedure. The vertebral artery can be detected by using the Doppler mode (Figure 12.4).

12.2.4 Practical block technique

Once the C4 root is detected at the top of the corresponding transverse process between the anterior and posterior tuberculi, the block is performed by using the OOP technique with the aim of positioning the tip of the needle dorsal to the root (Figure 12.5). This dorsal block technique has a certain protective effect, avoiding inadvertent slippage of the needle into an artery. The roots of nerves C2 and C3 roots are blocked in an analogue manner.

12.2.5 Essentials

Block characteristic	Advanced technique
Patient position	Supine, retroflexed, and slightly contralateral rotated neck
Ultrasound equipment	Linear probe, 25–38mm
Specific ultrasound setting	Maximum frequency of the probe
Important anatomical structures	C5 root, anterior and posterior tuberculi of the transverse process
Ultrasound appearance of the neuronal structures	Hypoechoic, round
Expected Vienna score	2
Needle equipment	50mm, Facette tip
Technique	OOP
Estimated local anaesthetic volume	2mL/root

12.3 Superficial cervical plexus blockade

12.3.1 Anatomy

The superficial cervical plexus forms the smaller occipital (from C2), greater auricular (from C2 and C3), cutaneous cervical (from C2 and C3), and supraclavicular (from C3 and C4) nerves.

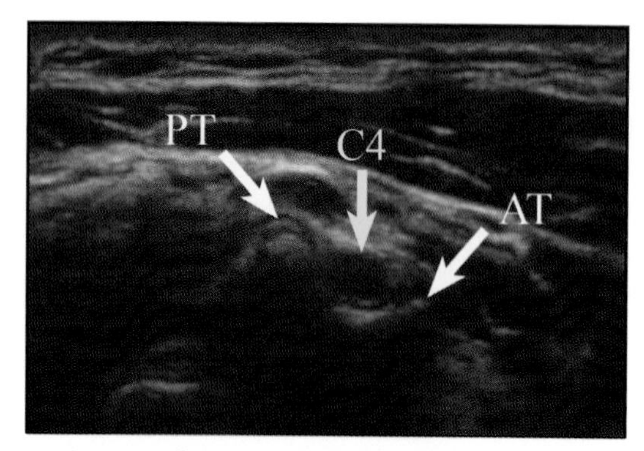

Fig. 12.2 Ultrasound image of the C4 root between the anterior and posterior tubercles of the C4 transverse process. AT: anterior tubercle; PT: posterior tubercle; right side=anterior.

The *smaller occipital nerve* curves around and ascends along the posterior border of the sternocleidomastoid muscle, supplies the skin behind the auricula, and communicates with the greater occipital and greater auricular nerves and the posterior auricular branch of the facial nerve.

The *greater auricular nerve* winds around the posterior border of the sternocleidomastoid muscle, ascending upon the muscle beneath the platysma to the parotid gland.

The *cutaneous (transverse) cervical nerve* turns around the posterior border of the sternocleidomastoid muscle and passes obliquely forward, beneath the

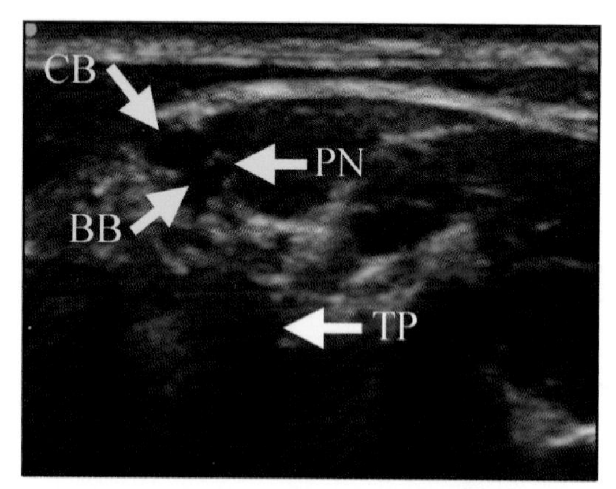

Fig. 12.3 Division of the C4 root into a cervical branch (CB), brachial branch (BB), and the phrenic nerve. CB: cervical branch; BB: brachial branch; PN: phrenic nerve; TP: transverse process; left side=anterior.

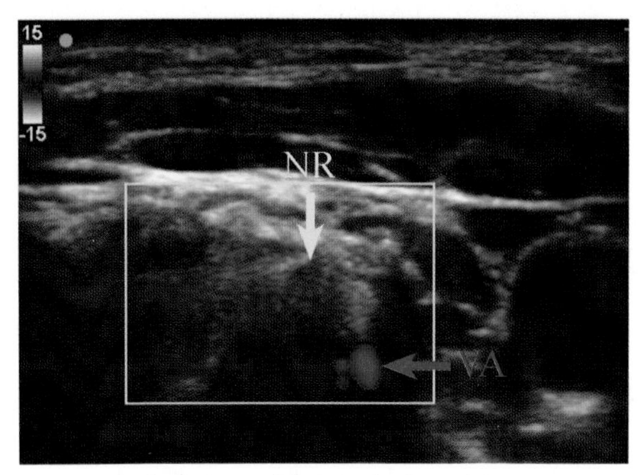

Fig. 12.4 Doppler mode illustration of the vertebral artery in close proximity to the nerve root. VA: vertebral artery; NR: nerve root; the quality of the NR image is attenuated to optimize the illustration of the VA; left side=anterior.

external jugular vein to the anterior border of the muscle to perforate the deep cervical fascia.

The *supraclavicular nerves* emerge beneath the posterior border of the sternocleidomastoid muscle and descend in the posterior triangle of the neck beneath the platysma and deep cervical fascia. Near the clavicle, the nerves become cutaneous and arrange into anterior, middle, and posterior parts.

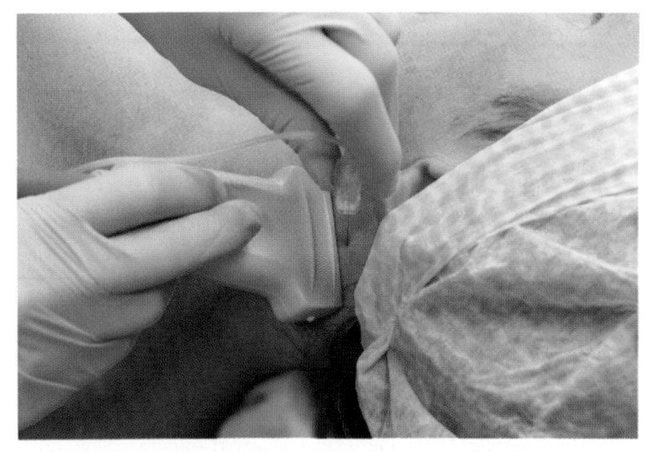

Fig. 12.5 OOP needle guidance technique for the C4 root blockade.
The C3 and C2 roots are equally blocked with slightly cranial probe and needle positions.

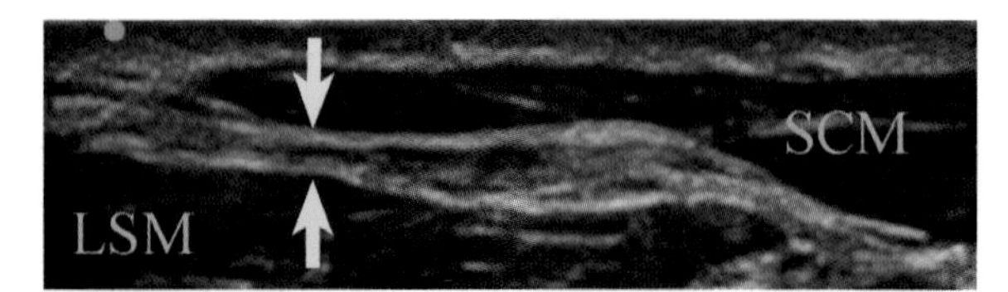

Fig. 12.6 Ultrasound image of the superficial cervical plexus (between the yellow arrows) behind the sternocleidomastoid muscle. SCM: sternocleidomastoid muscle; LSM: levator scapulae muscle; left side=posterior.

12.3.2 Ultrasound guidance technique

The superficial part of the cervical plexus can be visualized between the sternocleidomastoid and levator scapulae muscles, appearing oval and hyperechoic (Figure 12.6). An accurate identification of the individual parts of the superficial cervical plexus is theoretically possible, but too complex for daily clinical practice. The *greater auricular nerve* is one example where an individual nerve can be visualized where it winds around the sternocleidomastoid muscle as hypoechoic, oval-shaped nerve structures below the muscle and between the muscle and platysma (Figure 12.7).

12.3.3 Practical block technique

After the identification of the nerve structures between the sternocleidomastoid and levator scapulae muscles at a level slightly above the cricoid cartilage, the block should be performed using an IP technique as illustrated in Figures 12.8 and 12.9. The needle is advanced in the direction of the

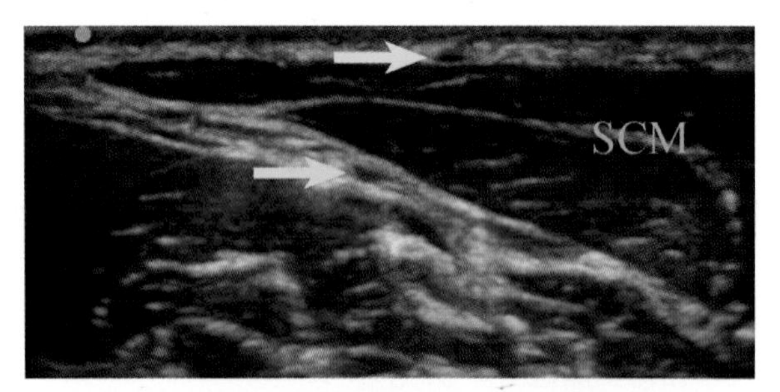

Fig. 12.7 The greater auricular nerve appears as a hypoechoic nerve structure and can be optimally visualized via ultrasound when it winds around the sternocleidomastoid muscle. SCM: sternocleidomastoid muscle; yellow arrows: subcutaneous and submuscular position of the greater auricular nerve; left side=posterior.

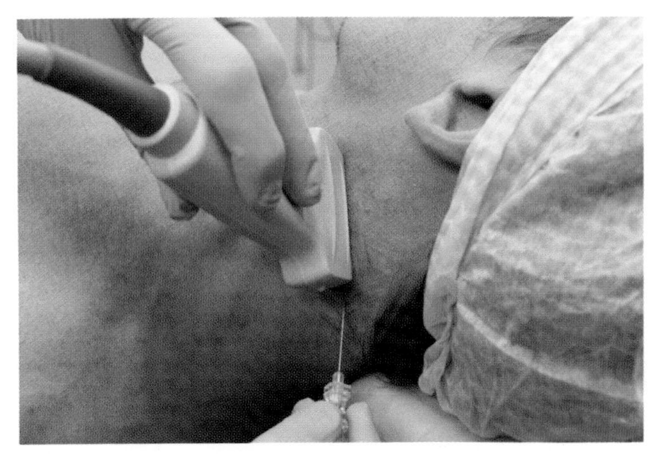

Fig. 12.8 IP position of the needle relative to the ultrasound probe for the superficial cervical plexus blockade.

carotid artery. The spread of local anaesthetic follows the fascial space below the sternocleidomastoid muscle until it reaches the carotid sheath. Ultrasonographic identification of the carotid artery is a prerequisite for a safe performance of this technique.

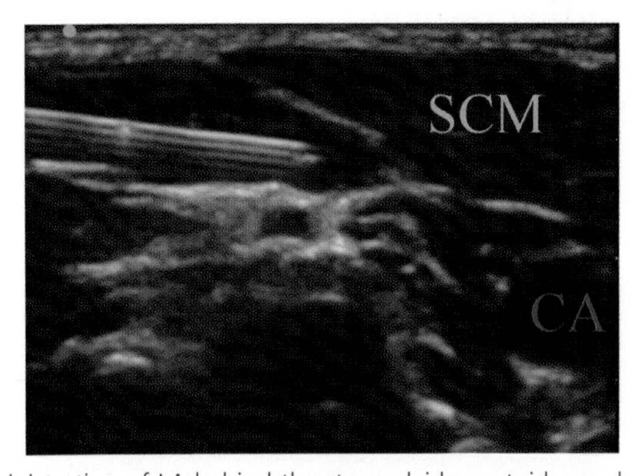

Fig. 12.9 Administration of LA behind the sternocleidomastoid muscle for the superficial cervical plexus blockade. SCM: sternocleidomastoid muscle; CA: carotid artery; left side=posterior.

12.3.4 Essentials

Block characteristic	Basic technique
Patient position	Supine, neck slightly rotated to the contralateral side
Ultrasound equipment	Linear probe, 38mm
Specific ultrasound setting	Maximum frequency of the probe
Important anatomical structures	Sternocleidomastoid muscle, levator scapulae muscle, carotid artery
Ultrasound appearance of the neuronal structures	Hyperechoic, oval
Expected Vienna score	2–3
Needle equipment	50mm, Facette tip
Technique	IP
Estimated local anaesthetic volume	2–4mL

12.4 Implication of neck blocks in children

The *superficial cervical plexus blockade* is useful in children as an adjunct to general anaesthesia for the ear and as part of the regional anaesthetic concept for head surgery (where in specific cases, the supraorbital, supratrochlear, infraorbital, or greater occipital nerves need to be blocked). The ultrasound-guided technique for superficial cervical plexus blockade is exactly the same as in adults. In children under 6 years old, a smaller probe (25mm) and the use of a 24–25G needle can be recommended.

Suggested further reading

Thallaj, A., Marhofer, P., Moriggl, B., Delvi, B.M., Kettner, S.C., Almajed, M., (2010). Great auricular nerve blockade via high resolution ultrasound: A volunteer study. *Anaesthesia*: in press.

Chapter 13

Upper extremity blocks

13.1 General anatomical considerations

The brachial plexus is formed by the ventral rami of the spinal nerves C5–T1. In general, supraclavicular and infraclavicular parts are described. The ventral rami leave the intervertebral foramina posterior to the vertebral artery and after a short distance in the scalenovertebral triangle (bordered by the longus colli muscle medially, the anterior scalenus muscle laterally, and the dome of the pleura inferiorly), they are situated between the anterior and middle scalene muscles (the interscalene space). The first branches are the *dorsal scapular* and *thoracic longus nerves,* both of which pierce the middle scalenus muscle to take a dorsolateral course. Subsequently, the roots form a superior (C5/C6), intermediate (C7), and inferior (C8/T1) trunk.

The third branch in the lateral cervical region is the *supraclavicular nerve* which shows a variable level of origin out of the superior trunk. Between the level of the first rib and the clavicle, each trunk bifurcates into an anterior and posterior portion to be rearranged and form the three cords of the brachial plexus. A lateral cord is formed by the anterior portion of the superior and middle trunks, a medial cord by the anterior portion of the inferior trunk, and a posterior cord by the posterior portions of all three trunks. The nomenclature of the three cords (lateral, medial, and posterior) refers to their position around the axillary artery. Note that their respective positions are different in the infraclavicular region (clavipectoral triangle) where they are situated laterally to the artery. The most superficial one is the lateral cord, followed by the posterior and medial cord as the deepest.

The brachial plexus is covered by connective tissue from its origin down to the axillary level. Various septae between the cords and nerves of the plexus appear to be responsible for incomplete nerve blockade, particularly at the axillary level when single-injection techniques are used.

13.2 **Interscalene brachial plexus approach**

13.2.1 Anatomy

The interscalene groove is bordered by the anterior scalenus muscle medially, the middle scalenus muscle laterally, and the first rib inferiorly (Figure 13.1). Its location is approximately beneath the lateral border of the sternocleidomastoid muscle when the head is rotated to the opposite side. Of note, the interscalene groove is covered more or less by the sternocleidomastoid muscle in the case of a neutral head position. The scalene muscles and the brachial plexus are covered by the prevertebral layer of the cervical fascia. Figure 13.2 illustrates the ultrasound anatomy of the brachial plexus at the level of the interscalene groove.

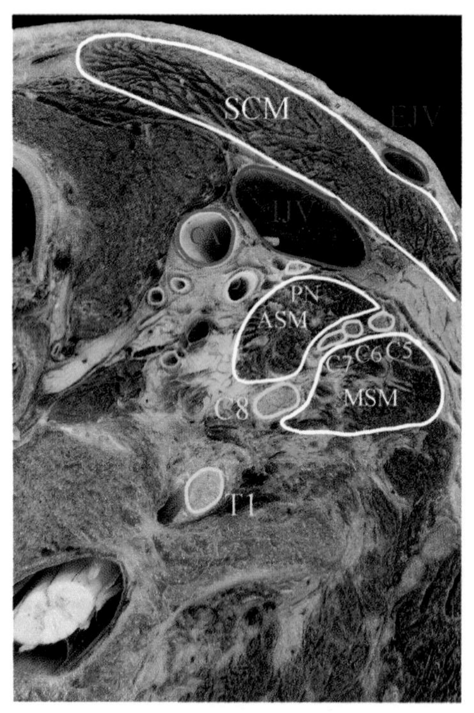

Fig. 13.1 Anatomical cross-sectional image of the nerve roots of the brachial plexus (C5–T1) inside the posterior interscalene groove. SCM: sternocleidomastoid muscle; ASM: anterior scalene muscle; MSM: middle scalene muscle; PN: phrenic nerve; CA: carotid artery; IJV: internal jugular vein; EJA: external jugular vein; left side=medial.

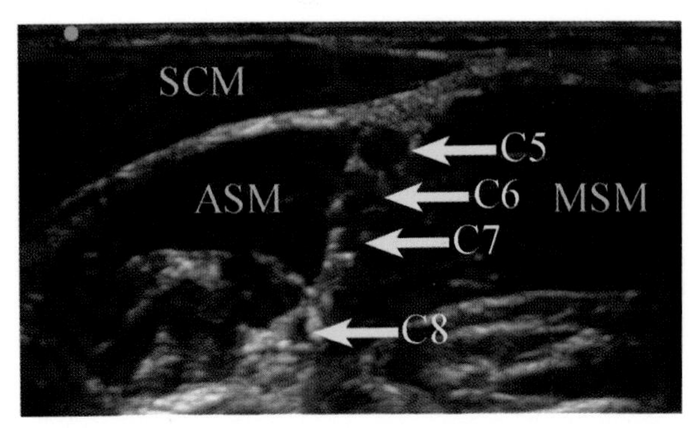

Fig. 13.2 Ultrasound image of the posterior interscalene groove.The C5–8 nerve roots are located lateral to the sternocleidomastoid muscle (SCM) and between the anterior (ASM) and median scalene muscles (MSM); left side=medial.

13.2.2 Anatomical variations

The brachial plexus often receives a communication from the ventral ramus C4. In this case, the plexus is situated more cephalic in relation to the cervical spine and designated as high or *prefixed*. In prefixed plexuses, C4 provides a large branch and the ventral ramus T1 appears small. When receiving the majority of communications from the ventral ramus C5, the brachial plexus is located more caudally and considered to be low or *postfixed*. In postfixed plexuses, the ventral ramus of T1 is large with an additional branch to the plexus provided by T2.

Variants of the course of the brachial plexus and its components have also been described. In a significant number of cases, the nerve roots are located medial (close to the greater vessels of the neck) or lateral to the lateral border of the sternocleidomastoid muscle. The C5–C7 roots may pierce the anterior scalenus muscle either together or separately (Figure 13.3). In some cases, only C5 pierces the anterior scalenus. These situations were found to occur unilaterally or bilaterally to the same extent. In a smaller number of cases, the C5 root may be found completely anterior to the anterior scalenus muscle (Figure 13.4). A scalenus minimus muscle may be present which is visualized as a small muscle slip running anterior to one or two of the roots. In a significant number of cases, a muscle bridge is located between the C7 and C8 roots (Figure 13.5). In rare cases, the subclavian artery has been found to pierce the anterior scalenus muscle with an accompanying post-stenotic dilatation. The dorsal scapular artery (former transversa colli) may arise from the subclavian artery more medially and take an ascending course between the roots. Muscular tissue interposed between the roots is a frequent finding.

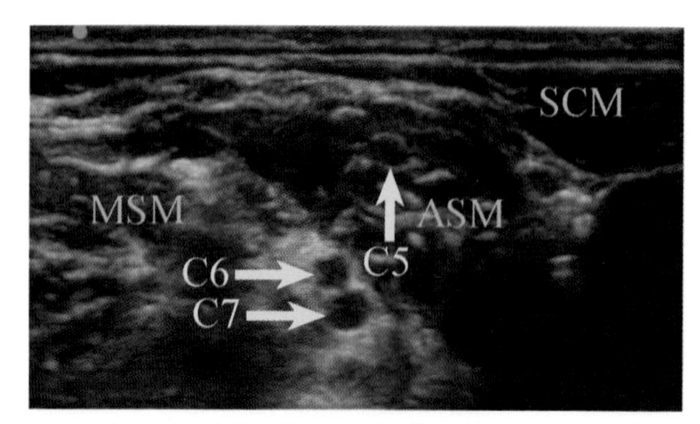

Fig. 13.3 Ultrasound image of the C5 root piercing the anterior scalene muscle (ASM).The C6 and 7 roots are located between the ASM and the median scalene muscles (MSM). SCM: sternocleidomastoid muscle; left side=lateral.

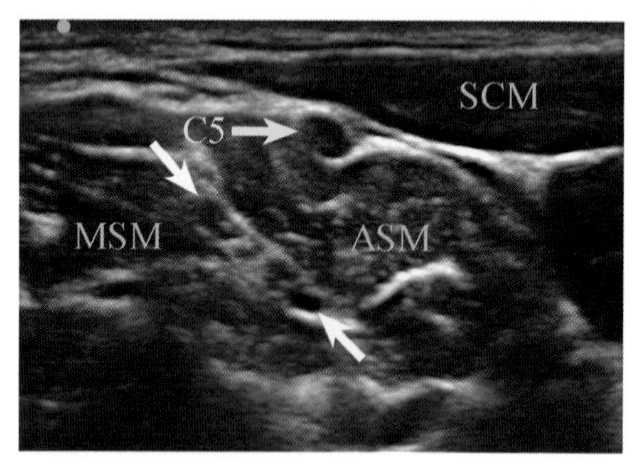

Fig. 13.4 Ultrasound image of the C5 root anterior to the anterior scalene muscle (ASM) and completely outside the posterior interscalene groove (white arrows). SCM: sternocleidomastoid muscle; MSM: middle scalene muscle; left side=lateral.

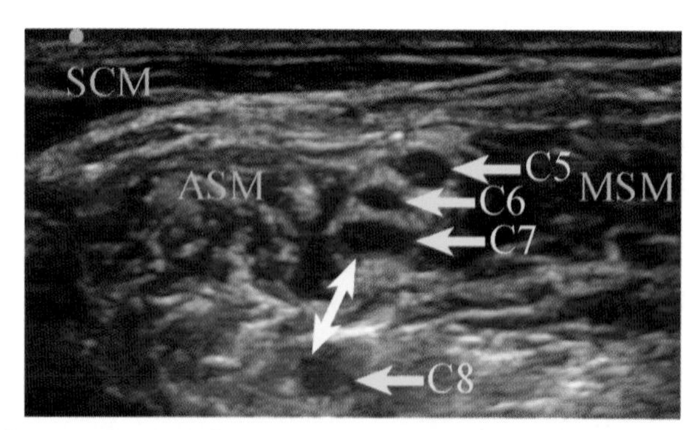

Fig. 13.5 Ultrasound image of a typical muscle bridge (white arrow) between the C7 and C8 roots.The C5–7 roots are already surrounded by local anaesthetic. SCM: sternocleidomastoid muscle; ASM: anterior scalene muscle; MSM: middle scalene muscle; left side=medial.

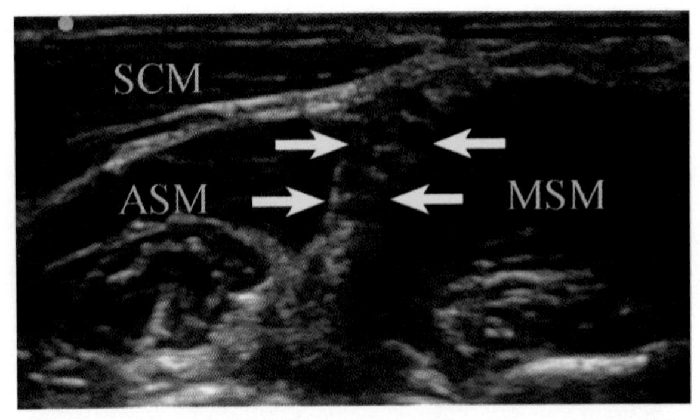

Fig. 13.6 Ultrasound image of the bifurcations of the nerve roots inside the posterior interscalene groove as the scanning head is slightly laterally moved from the initial position when the nerve roots are visualized as illustrated in Figure 13.2.
SCM: sternocleidomastoid muscle; ASM: anterior scalene muscle; MSM: middle scalene muscle; left side=medial.

13.2.3 Ultrasound guidance technique

Ultrasound investigation starts at the middle of the neck, at the level where the larynx is most prominent and the greater vessels of the neck are easy visible. Thereafter, the probe is moved slowly in a lateral direction up to the lateral border of the sternocleidomastoid muscle. Once the lateral border of the sternocleidomastoid muscle and the anterior and middle scalene muscles are visible, the position of the probe relative to the skin should be slightly moved from a perpendicular to a caudally oblique direction. The nerve roots appear between the anterior and middle scalene muscles inside the posterior interscalene groove as round or oval hypoechoic structures (Figure 13.2). When scanned more distally, the bifurcations may be visualized (Figure 13.6).

13.2.4 Practical block technique

It should be taken into consideration that the external jugular vein is usually visible in the final probe position. The puncture site should therefore be chosen medial or lateral to the external jugular vein.

The needle direction relative to the position of the probe should be OOP from cranial (Figure 13.7). Taking a posterior approach using the IP technique can lead to the potential disadvantage of the needle moving perpendicularly to the interscalene groove. As mentioned above, the *dorsal scapular* and *thoracic longus nerves* pierce the middle scalenus muscle as the first branches of the brachial plexus (Figure 13.8). They provide motor supply to the shoulder girdle and should be considered at risk if the IP technique is used in a posterior approach through the middle scalenus muscle. Thus, the OOP technique is the anatomically preferential method. Following the positioning of the needle tip between the nerve structures and the anterior and middle scalene muscles, the

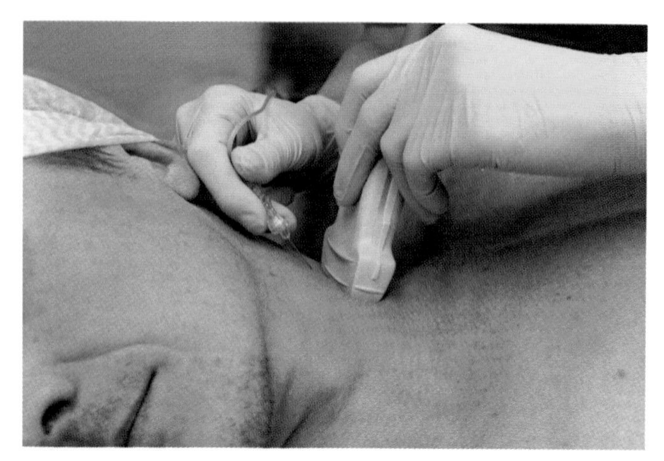

Fig. 13.7 OOP position of the needle relative to the ultrasound probe for the interscalene block technique.

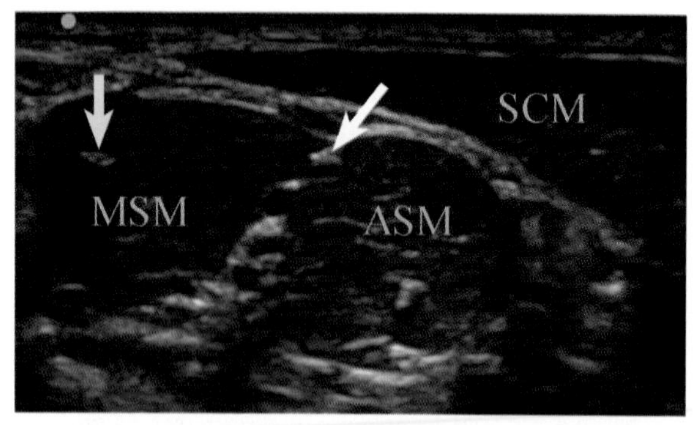

Fig. 13.8 Ultrasound image of a nerve structure (yellow arrow) inside the middle scalene muscle.The white arrow indicates the nerve roots inside the posterior interscalene groove. SCM: sternocleidomastoid muscle; MSM: middle scalene muscle; ASM: anterior scalene muscle; left side=lateral.

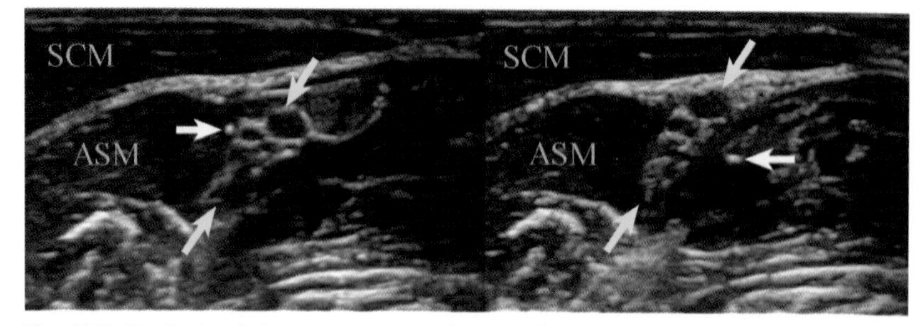

Fig. 13.9 Blockade of the nerve roots with a needle position medial (left side of the figure) and lateral (right side of the figure) to the neuronal structures (located between the yellow arrows). The local anaesthetic appears hypoechoic.
SCM: sternocleidomastoid muscle; ASM: anterior scalene muscle; left side=medial.

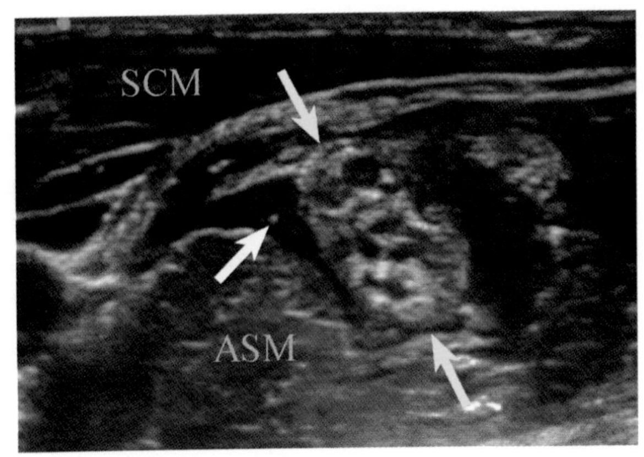

Fig. 13.10 Typical appearance of connective tissue around nerve roots (between the yellow arrows) after administration of local anaesthetic. The white arrow indicates the tip of the needle. SCM: sternocleidomastoid muscle; ASM: anterior scalene muscle; left side=medial.

local anaesthetic is administered (Figure 13.9). Depending on the spread of the anaesthetic, redirection of the needle to a position between the nerve structures and the anterior scalene muscle may be necessary. If a muscle bridge is detected between the C7 and C8 root or if blockade of the T1 root is required, it is necessary to adjust the depth of the needle. In these cases, care should be taken to avoid an inadvertent neuraxial position of the needle tip. After administration of the local anaesthetic by the described multi-injection technique, the nerve roots are much better presentable on ultrasound (a general rule for most of regional anaesthetic techniques). In addition, connective tissue can be identified, which could influence onset times (Figure 13.10). The quantity of connective tissue between the local anaesthetic and the neuronal structures do not influence the success rates of individual blocks.

13.2.5 Essentials

Block characteristic	Basic technique
Patient position	Supine, arm adducted, elbow slightly flexed
Ultrasound equipment	Linear probe, 38mm
Specific ultrasound setting	Maximum frequency of the probe
Important anatomical structures	Sternocleidomastoid muscle, anterior and middle scalene muscles
Ultrasound appearance of the neuronal structures	Round or oval, hypoechoic
Expected Vienna score	1–2
Needle equipment	50mm, Facette tip
Technique	OOP
Estimated local anaesthetic volume	8–12mL

13.3 Supraclavicular approach

13.3.1 Anatomy

In the supraclavicular region, between the first rib and the clavicle, the brachial plexus becomes rearranged as described in Section 13.1 (Figure 13.11). The plexus is located laterally to the subclavian artery which is situated close to the pleura and the first rib (Figure 13.12). If present, the dorsal scapular artery (former transverse colli) arises from the subclavian artery and traverses the brachial plexus regularly (Figure 13.13).

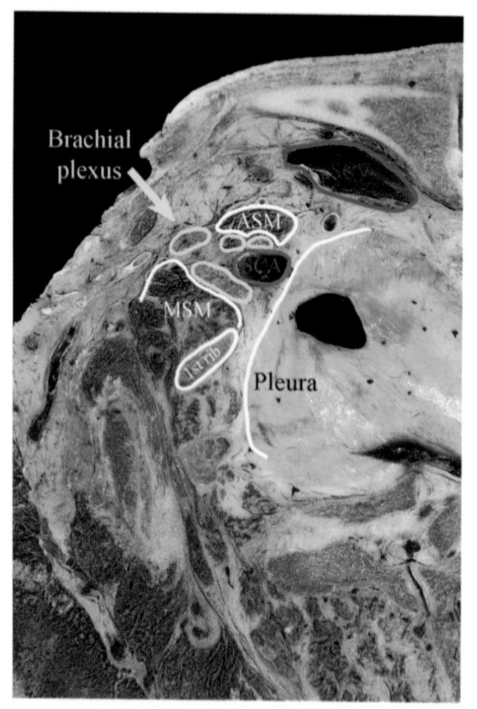

Fig. 13.11 Anatomical cross-sectional image of the brachial plexus in the supraclavicular region. ASM: anterior scalene muscle; MSM: middle scalene muscle; SCA: subclavian artery; SCV: subclavian vein; left side=lateral.

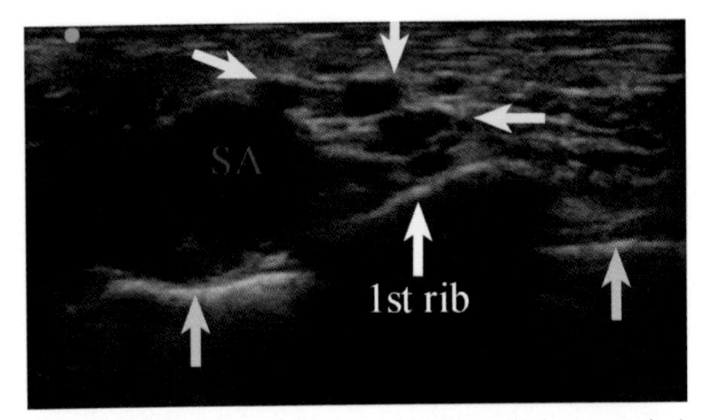

Fig. 13.12 Ultrasound illustration of the brachial plexus in the supraclavicular region lateral to the subclavian artery and above the 1st rib. The grey arrows indicate the cervical pleura. The nerve structures appear as hypoechoic, round and oval structures and are labelled between the yellow arrows. SA: subclavian artery; left side=medial.

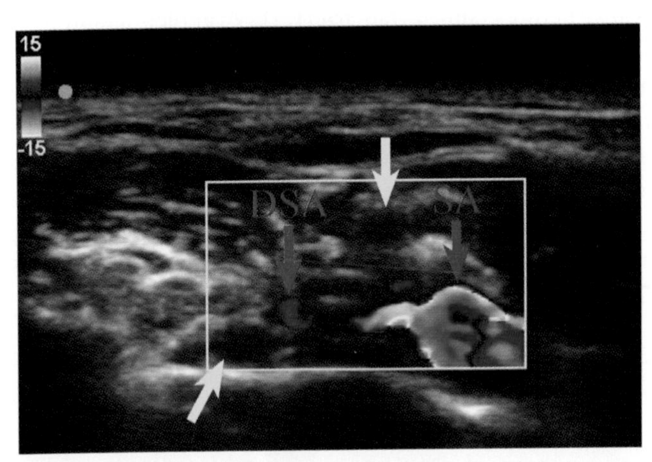

Fig. 13.13 A dorsal suprascapular artery may arise from the subclavian artery and traverses the brachial plexus in the supraclavicular region. The yellow arrows mark parts of the brachial plexus. DSA: dorsal suprascapular artery; SA: subclavian artery; left side=lateral.

13.3.2 Anatomical variations

If the dorsal scapular artery has a more prominent appearance than expected, an infraclavicular approach should be considered (see Section 13.4). It should also be noted that the *suprascapular nerve* has a variable level of origin from the superior trunk (see Section 13.6).

13.3.3 Ultrasound guidance technique

Ultrasound investigation should start as described for the interscalene approach (see Section 13.2). Once the brachial plexus is adequately identified within the interscalene space, a further caudal movement of the probe allows the identification of the neural structures as multiple, round and oval hypoechoic structures lateral to the subclavian artery (Figure 13.12). The anterior and middle scalene muscles can be traced distally to their insertion on the first rib.

13.3.4 Practical block technique

Once the nerve structures of the brachial plexus and all the relevant adjacent anatomical structures (subclavian artery, cervical pleura, and first rib) are identified, an IP technique should be used with a needle insertion site from the posterior (Figures 13.14 and 13.15). After careful aspiration and initial administration of a small volume of local anaesthetic, an intermediate analysis of the spread of fluid is mandatory. If the spread is regular, the needle position can be maintained and local anaesthetic should be administered until all nerve structures are surrounded. If the initial needle position does not give a regular spread, the needle should be repositioned. Sometimes, a number of needle positions are necessary.

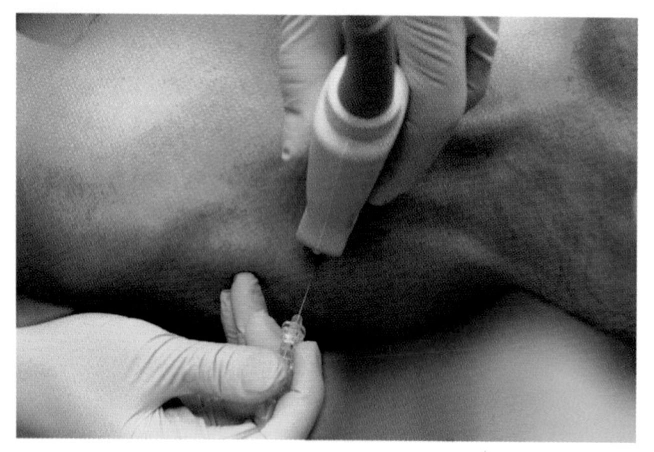

Fig. 13.14 IP needle guidance technique for the supraclavicular brachial plexus block technique with a posterior–medial needle direction.

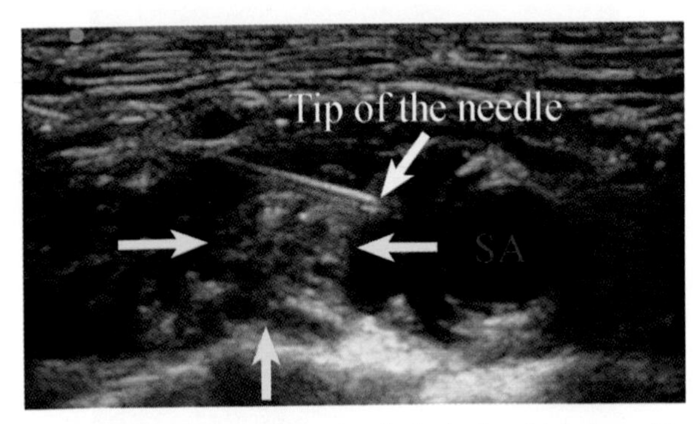

Fig. 13.15 Ultrasound illustration of a supraclavicular brachial plexus blockade with an IP needle guidance technique. The neuronal structures are labelled with the yellow arrows. The anechoic areas around the neuronal structures represent the local anaesthetic. SA: subclavian artery; left side=lateroposterior.

13.3.5 Essentials

Block characteristic	Intermediate technique
Patient position	Supine, arm adducted, elbow slightly flexed, neck slightly retroflexed (pillow under shoulders)
Ultrasound equipment	Linear probe, 25 or 38mm
Specific ultrasound setting	Maximum frequency of the probe
Important anatomical structures	Anterior and median scalene muscles, subclavian muscle, subclavian artery, cervical pleura, first rib
Ultrasound appearance of the neuronal structures	Round and oval hypoechoic
Expected Vienna score	1–2
Needle equipment	50mm, Facette tip
Technique	IP
Estimated local anaesthetic volume	8–10mL

13.4 Infraclavicular approach

13.4.1 Anatomy

The three cords of the brachial plexus (see Section 13.1) enter the infraclavicular region at the clavipectoral triangle lateral to the axillary artery and vein (Figure 13.16). The cephalic vein, which varies in size, crosses the brachial plexus superficially.

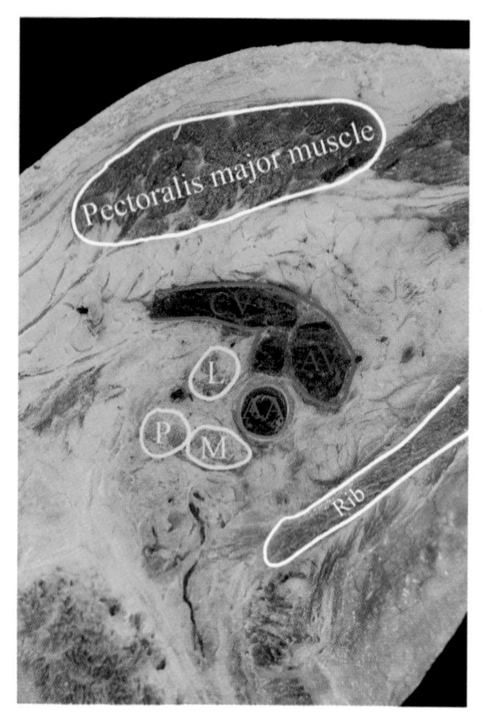

Fig. 13.16 Anatomical cross-sectional image of the brachial plexus in the infraclavicular region. L: lateral cord; M: medial cord; P: posterior cord; CV: cephalic vein; AV: axillary vein; AA: axillary artery; left side=lateral.

13.4.2 Anatomical variations

The medial and lateral or the medial and posterior cords may be present as a common cord. Rare cases of a single cord have been described. The most common minor variants are related to the position of the cords around the artery.

13.4.3 Ultrasound guidance technique

The position of the ultrasound probe should be 30–45° oblique relative to the clavicle. Using a linear probe at medium frequencies (10MHz), the subclavian artery is visualized as a round structure and the cords of the brachial plexus as hyperechoic round structures (Figure 13.17). In cases of significant muscle masses above the nerve structures (pectoralis major and minor muscles), the optimal visualization of the nerve structures may be impaired. Nevertheless, the medial and lateral cords constantly remain below the fascia of the pectoralis minor muscle. In some cases, an adequate visualization of the posterior cord might be difficult.

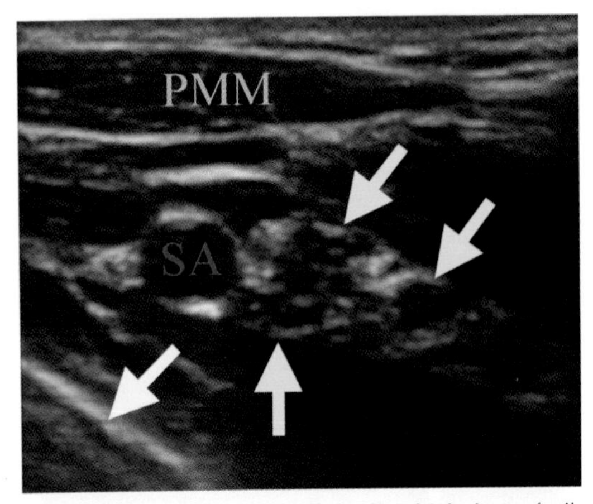

Fig. 13.17 Ultrasound image of the cords of the brachial plexus (yellow arrows) in the infraclavicular region lateral to the subclavian artery and below the pectoralis major muscle. The white arrow indicates the pleura. SA: subclavian artery; PMM: pectoralis major muscle; left side=medial.

13.4.4 Practical block technique

An OOP technique should be used with a needle position from above or below the probe (Figure 13.18). Once the needle is placed lateral to the subclavian artery and below the pectoralis minor muscle, the local anaesthetic can be administered after careful aspiration. A spread lateral to and below the artery provides an optimal block result (Figure 13.19).

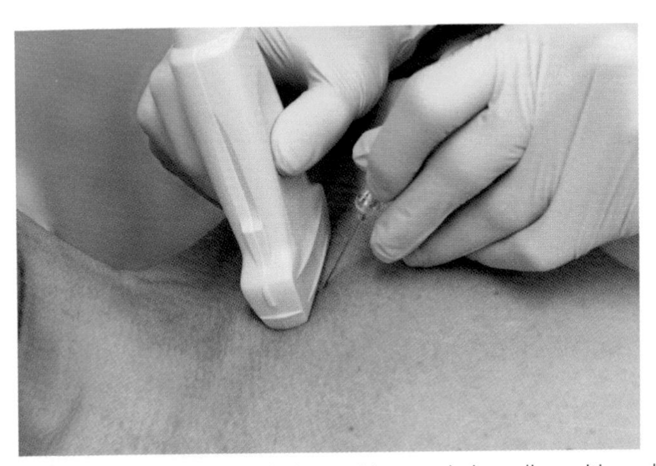

Fig. 13.18 OOP needle guidance technique with a caudad needle position relative to the ultrasound probe.

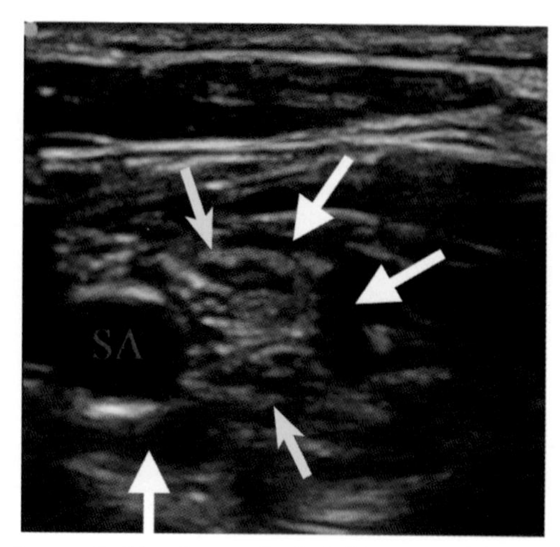

Fig. 13.19 Correct spread of local anaesthetic (white arrows) in a lateral and caudal direction relative to the cords (yellow arrows). SA: subclavian artery; left side=medial.

13.4.5 Essentials

Block characteristic	Intermediate technique
Patient position	Supine, arm adducted, elbow slightly flexed
Ultrasound equipment	Linear probe, 38mm
Specific ultrasound setting	Medium frequency of the probe
Important anatomical structures	Subclavian artery, pectoralis major and minor muscles, pleura
Ultrasound appearance of the neuronal structures	Round, hyperechoic
Expected Vienna score	2–3
Needle equipment	50mm, Facette tip
Technique	OOP
Estimated local anaesthetic volume	8–15mL

13.5 Axillary approach

13.5.1 Anatomy

The following anatomical description (Figure 13.20) is based upon a probe position as illustrated in Figure 13.21 where the left side of the image is orientated

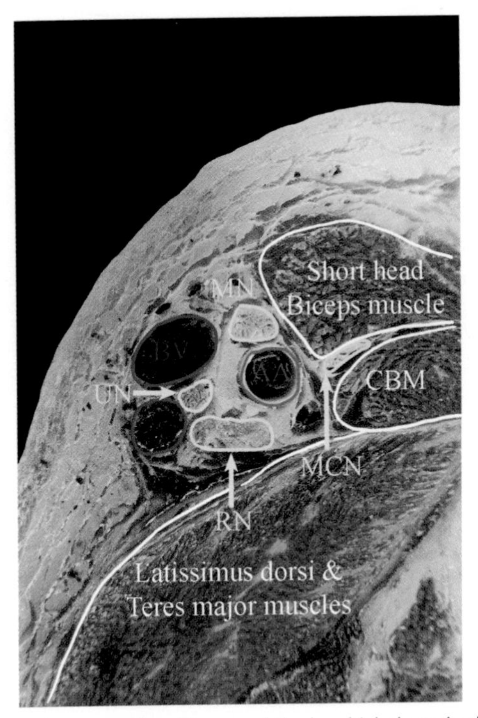

Fig. 13.20 Anatomical cross-sectional image of the brachial plexus in the axillary region. MN: median nerve; RN: radial nerve; UN: ulnar nerve; MCN: musculocutaneous nerve; BV: basilic vein; AA: axillary artery; CBM: coracobrachialis muscle.

to the anterior surface of the upper arm. The major branches of the brachial plexus are arranged around the axillary artery in a variable manner. As the most superficial branch, the median nerve is usually found in a 10 to 12 o'clock position in relation to the artery. The ulnar nerve is usually in a 2 to 4 o'clock position, but the distance to the artery varies. In a significant number of cases, the basilic vein is interposed between the axillary artery and the ulnar nerve. The radial nerve lies below the artery in a 3 to 6 o'clock position. The musculocutaneous nerve originates more proximally from the lateral cord at the level of the coracoid process and usually pierces the coracobrachialis muscle. The medial brachial and medial antebrachial cutaneous nerves are situated superficially beneath the brachial fascia and their visualization is not always feasible. The brachial artery, together with the median, ulnar, and radial nerves, form a neurovascular bundle that is enveloped by the so-called axillary sheath which is derived from the prevertebral layer of the cervical fascia. Numerous septae attached to the inner surface of the axillary sheath divide the neurovascular bundle, providing variable compartments for each nerve.

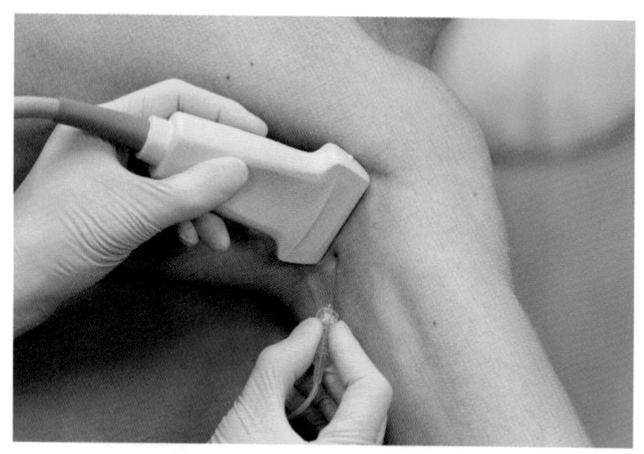

Fig. 13.21 OOP needle guidance technique for axillary brachial plexus blockade.

13.5.2 Anatomical variations

The most frequent variants encountered in the axilla are the positions of the four nerves around the axillary artery. The site of formation of the median nerve (i.e. the union of the medial and lateral branches) has been found as far down as the cubita. The median nerve or its branches may also pass behind the artery.

The musculocutaneous nerve typically runs behind the coracobrachialis muscle or between the coracobrachialis muscle and the short biceps head. Often, instead of piercing the coracobrachialis muscle, the nerves take a distal course, together with the median nerve, to pass between the biceps and brachialis muscles. Occasionally, only a portion of the nerve follows this course while the main branch pierces the coracobrachialis muscle as usual, subsequently fusing with the aberrant branch. A communicating branch from the median nerve has been described. In some cases, the median nerve may be doubled, unusually short, or even absent.

The radial nerve may join the axillary nerve and pass posteriorly to the humerus. In rare cases, the radial nerve may be absent whereupon the musculocutaneous and ulnar nerves take over its area of supply.

Note that veins may be present in various numbers and diameters.

13.5.3 Ultrasound guidance technique

Due to the fact that all structures in the axilla are in close proximity, it is not always possible to precisely analyze individual nerves using a single and static probe position. Tracking of the nerves facilitates their safe identification. When the axillary artery is scanned from the axillary level in a distal direction,

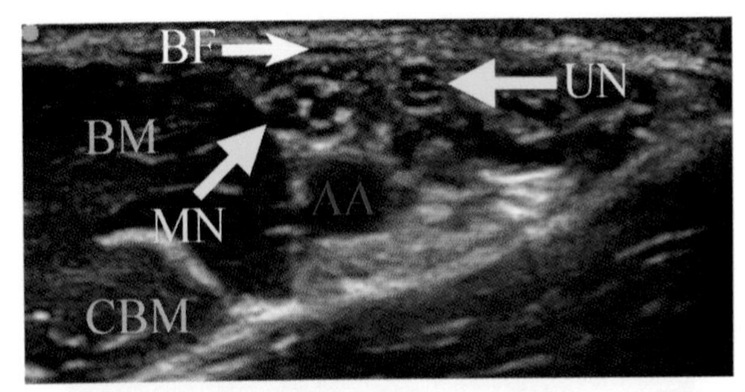

Fig. 13.22 Ultrasound illustration of the median and ulnar nerves at the level of the axilla. The visualization of the radial nerves (usually in a 4 to 6 o´clock position relative to the axillary artery) requires careful probe adjustment. MN: median nerve; UN: ulnar nerve; AA: axillary artery; BF: brachial fascia; BM: biceps muscle; CBM: coracobrachialis muscle; left side=cranial.

the *median nerve* is usually found close to the artery. The *ulnar nerve* can easily be identified as the most superficial nerve and passes beneath the brachial fascia distally to the level of the medial epicondyle. The *radial nerve* can be tracked from the sulcus of the radial nerve in a proximal direction where it usually lies in a position between the axillary artery and the medial head of the triceps muscle. It is important to state that the illustration of all three main nerves in one figure is extremely difficult and even in the best case, the illustration of the radial nerve is impaired. Figure 13.22 illustrates the location of the ulnar and median nerves.

By slightly moving the probe from the initial axillary position into a more oblique position, it is possible to visualize the musculocutaneous nerve as a triangular or oval and hyperechoic structure between the short head of the biceps muscle and the coracobrachial muscle (Figure 13.23).

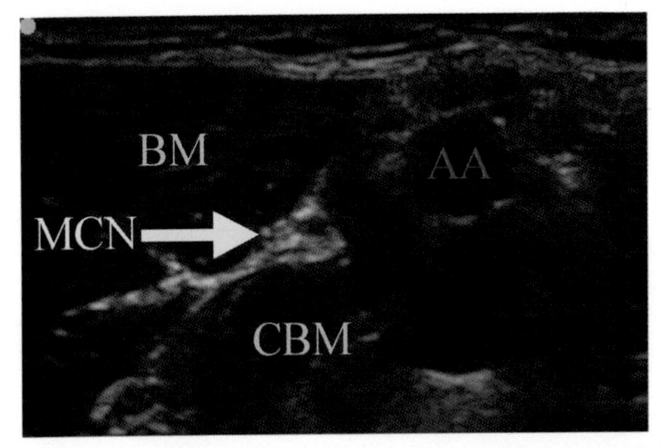

Fig. 13.23 The musculocutaneous nerve (MCN) between the biceps and the coracobrachialis muscles. BM: biceps muscle; CBM: coracobrachialis muscle; AA: axillary artery; left side=cranial.

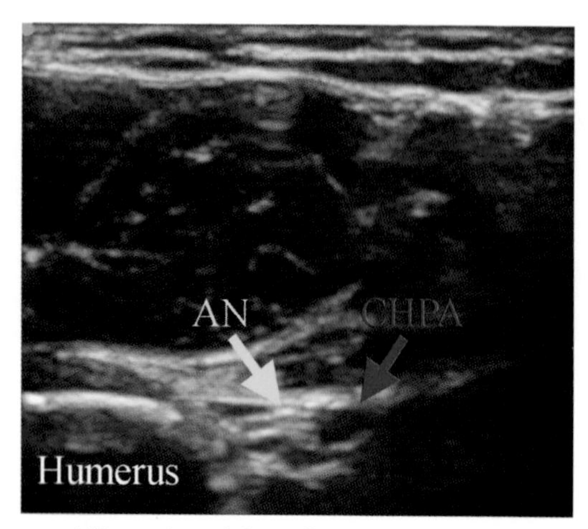

Fig. 13.24 Ultrasound illustration of the axillary nerve between the circumflexa humeri posterior artery and the humerus. AN: axillary nerve; CHPA: circumflexa humeri posterior artery; left side=cranial.

The probe position described above also enables the location of the axillary nerve (see Figure 13.24). By changing the settings to slightly lower frequencies, the pulsation of the circumflexa humeri posterior artery between the teres major and triceps muscles is possible. The axillary nerve lies in close proximity to that artery.

13.5.4 **Practical block technique**

After precisely locating the nerves in the axillary region, an OOP technique is indicated for the approach. The needle insertion site should be caudal to

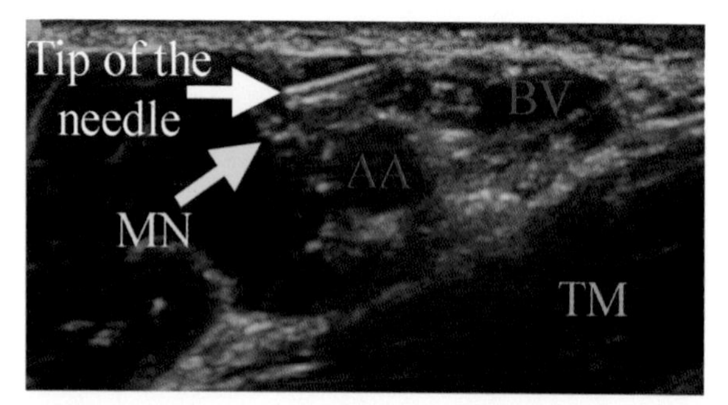

Fig. 13.25 Blockade of the median nerve during axillary brachial plexus blockade. MN: median nerve; AA: axillary artery; BV: basilic vein; TM: triceps muscle; left side=cranial.

the axillary artery in order to avoid muscle puncture. We recommend blocking the deeper structures first and then the more superficial structures. In case of air bubble-related artefacts (which can always occur no matter how well the technique is performed), the visibility below the relevant structures is impaired. The radial nerve should therefore be blocked first, followed by the ulnar, median, and musculocutaneous nerves by a multi-injection technique (Figures 13.25). Finally, the cutaneous branches of the medial cord should be blocked by the administration of a small volume of local anaesthetic beneath the brachial fascia (Figure 13.22).

Care should be taken to avoid an inadvertent intravascular position the needle. If the contact pressure of the ultrasound probe is suboptimal, the veins can disappear from the ultrasound image and the intravenous needle position cannot be detected either by direct visualization or by aspiration. The contact pressure of the probe should therefore be carefully adjusted to ensure that vein visibility (Figure 13.26).

The injection site described above also permits the blockade of the axillary nerve. Due to the depth of the axillary nerve and the need for a lower ultrasound resolution, the nerve is not as clearly visible as the more superficial nerves in that area. Care has to be taken to avoid an inadvertent puncture of the circumflexa humeri posterior artery.

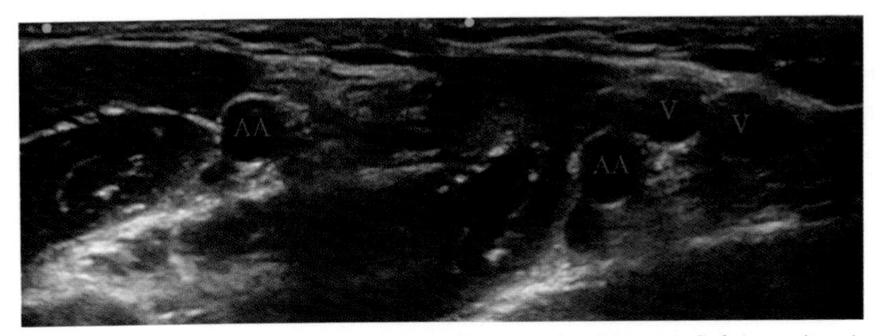

Fig. 13.26 Ultrasound illustrations of the axillary vessels with more (left image) and less (right image) probe pressure. The veins in the axillary area are easily compressible and disappear with too much pressure caused by the ultrasound probe. AA: axillary artery; V: vein; left side in both illustrations=cranial.

13.5.5 Essentials

Block characteristic	Basic technique
Patient position	Supine, arm 90° abducted
Ultrasound equipment	Linear probe, 38mm
Specific ultrasound setting	Maximum frequency of the probe
Important anatomical structures	Axillary artery and vein, basilic vein, circumflexa humeri posterior artery (as guidance structure of the axillary nerve), short head of the biceps muscle, coracobrachialis muscle, triceps muscle
Ultrasound appearance of the neuronal structures	Round and oval hyperechoic structures. The musculocutaneous nerve appears oval proximally and as a triangular hyperechoic structure more distally (between the upper and middle third of the humerus).
Expected Vienna score	1–2
Needle equipment	50mm, Facette tip
Technique	OOP
Estimated local anaesthetic volume	8–12mL

13.6 Suprascapular nerve block

13.6.1 Anatomy

The suprascapular nerve arises from the superior trunk and runs laterally beneath the trapezius and omohyoideus muscles. The nerve enters the supraspinatus fossa through the suprascapular notch below the superior transverse scapular ligament. It gives off branches to the supraspinatus and infraspinatus muscles and to the shoulder joint.

13.6.2 Anatomical variations

In some cases, the suprascapular nerve may divide into a superior and an inferior branch. The superior branch passes through or above the suprascapular notch while the inferior branch passes through a foramen below the suprascapular notch. The nerve has also been found to pass over the superior transverse scapular ligament.

13.6.3 Ultrasound guidance technique

With a scanning head position as described for the supraclavicular approach to the brachial plexus (Figure 13.12), the suprascapular nerve appears as a hypoechoic, round to slightly oval structure, running laterally when tracked from a proximal to distal position (Figure 13.27).

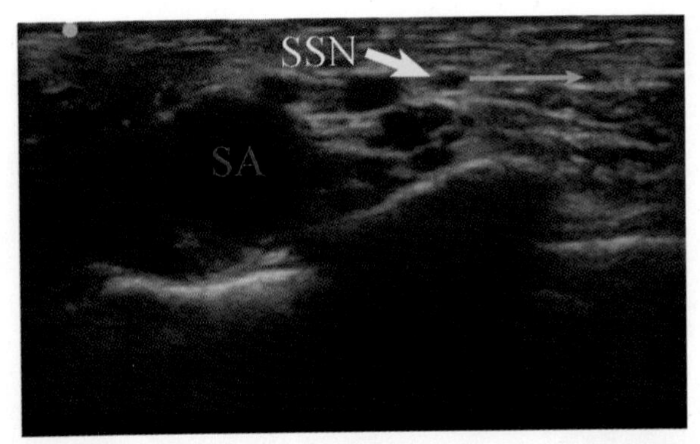

Fig. 13.27 Ultrasound image of the suprascapular nerve on its lateral course at the supraclavicular level.The grey arrow indicates the course of the nerve when the ultrasound probe is moved in a lateral direction. The hypoechoic round structures on the left side from the artery indicate the brachial plexus at the supraclavicular level. SSN: suprascapular nerve; SA: subclavian artery; left side=medial.

13.6.4 Practical block technique

The block should be performed using an IP technique with the probe in the position as described for the supraclavicular approach (Figure 13.14). A small volume (2mL) of local anaesthetic usually provides an adequate blockade of the suprascapular nerve.

13.6.5 Essentials

Block characteristic	Basic technique
Patient position	Supine, arm adducted, elbow slightly flexed, neck slightly retroflexed (pillow under shoulders)
Ultrasound equipment	Linear probe, 25 or 38mm
Specific ultrasound setting	Maximum frequency of the probe
Important anatomical structures	Anterior and median scalene muscles, subclavian muscle, subclavian artery, cervical pleura, first rib
Ultrasound appearance of the neuronal structures	Round and oval, hypoechoic structure
Expected Vienna score	1–2
Needle equipment	50mm, Facette tip
Technique	IP
Estimated local anaesthetic volume	2mL

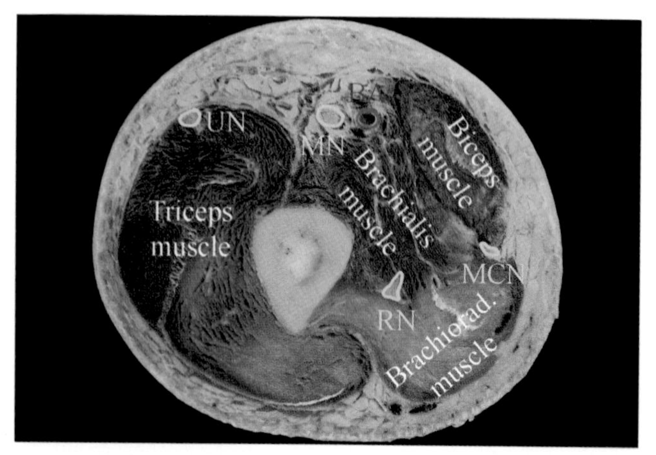

Fig. 13.28 Anatomical cross-sectional image of the peripheral nerves of the brachial plexus at the level of the distal upper arm. UN: ulnar nerve; MN: median nerve; RN: radial nerve; MCN: musculocutaneous nerve; BA: brachial artery; left side=ulnar.

13.7 **Median nerve block**

13.7.1 Anatomy

The median nerve is formed by parts of the lateral and medial cord on the anterior aspect of the brachial artery. It takes its course superficially to the brachial artery to enter the cubita. Subsequently, it usually passes between the humeral and ulnar heads of the pronator teres muscle. At the level of the proximal part of the forearm, the median nerve is embedded between the superficial and profound flexor digitorum muscles (Figures 13.28 and 13.29).

13.7.2 Anatomical variations

In a minority of cases, the median nerve may pierce the humeral head of the pronator teres muscle or lie between the ulnar head and ulna. The nerve has also been found to pass superficially on the surface of the flexor digitorum superficialis muscle. Some reports have observed that the median nerve may split into two branches in the forearm which pass through the carpal tunnel in separate compartments.

13.7.3 Ultrasound guidance technique

The echogenicity of the median nerve at the level of the cubita is moderate. More distally below the pronator teres muscle, the nerve is hardly visible whereas at the medial part of the forearm, between the superficial and

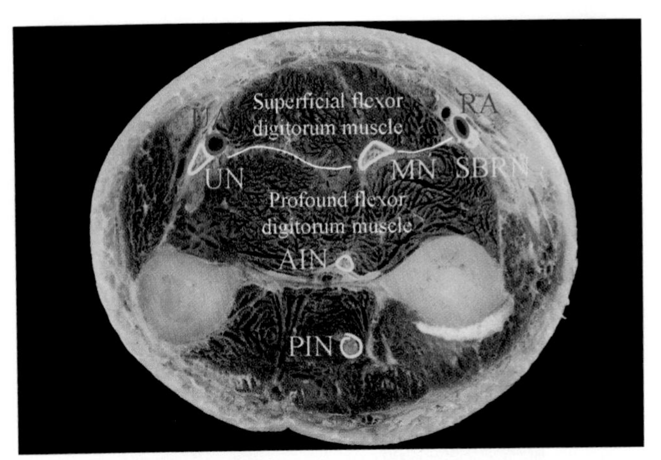

Fig. 13.29 Anatomical cross-sectional image of the peripheral nerves of the brachial plexus at the level of the mid-forearm. UN: ulnar nerve; MN: median nerve; SBRN: superficial branch of the radial nerve; AIN: anterior interosseous nerve; PIN: posterior interosseous nerve; RA: radial artery; UA: ulnar artery; left side=ulnar.

profound flexor digitorum muscles, it can be visualized clearly as a hyperechoic, round or oval structure (Figure 13.30).

13.7.4 Practical block technique

The median nerve should be blocked at the level between the superficial and profound flexor digitorum muscles. More proximally, where the nerve is in close proximity to the brachial artery and several fascial layers, blockade can be difficult due to the unpredictable spread of local anaesthetic. Using an OOP

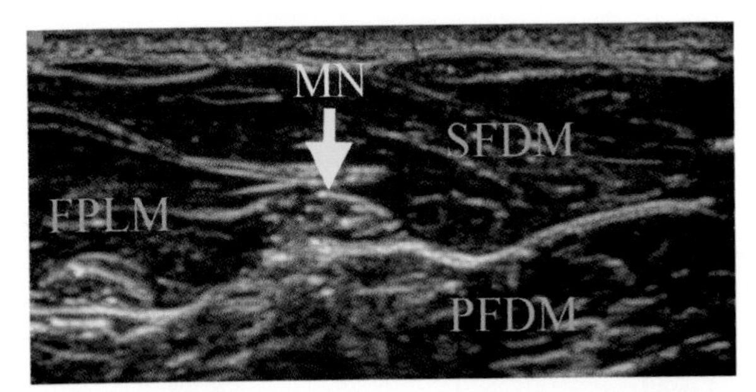

Fig. 13.30 Ultrasound image of the median nerve at the mid-forearm level between the superficial and profound flexor digitorum muscles. MN: median nerve; SFDM: superficial flexor digitorum muscle; PFDM: profound flexor digitorum muscle; FPLM: flexor pollicis longus muscle; left side=radial.

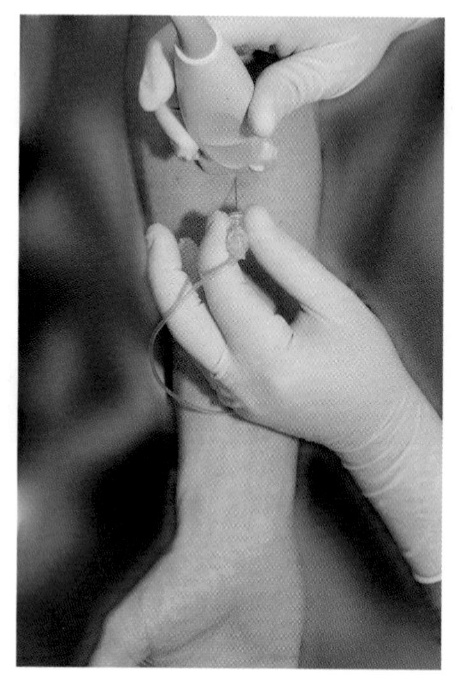

Fig. 13.31 OOP position of the probe relative to the needle for median nerve blockade at the level of the mid-forearm.

technique (Figure 13.31) with the needle between the superficial and profound flexor digitorum muscles in 3 and 9 o'clock positions, the nerve can be blocked with small volumes of local anaesthetic (Figure 13.32).

13.7.5 **Essentials**

Block characteristic	Basic technique
Patient position	Supine, arm slightly abducted, supinated position of the arm
Ultrasound equipment	Linear probe, 25–38mm
Specific ultrasound setting	Maximum frequency of the probe
Important anatomical structures	Superficial and profound flexor digitorum muscles
Ultrasound appearance of the neuronal structures	Hyperechoic (between the proximal and middle third of the forearm)
Expected Vienna score	1
Needle equipment	50mm, Facette tip
Technique	OOP
Estimated local anaesthetic volume	2mL

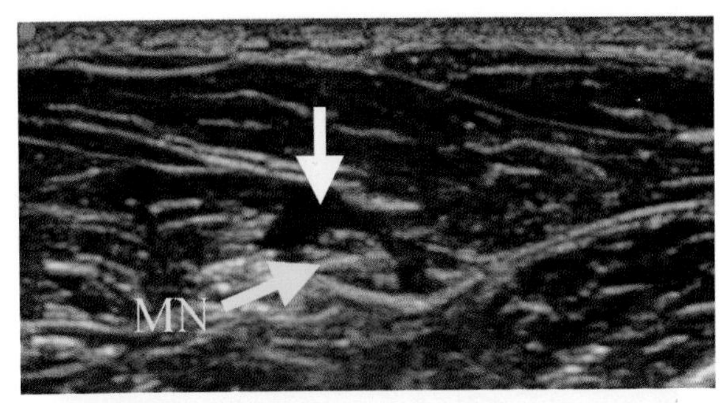

Fig. 13.32 The median nerve (MN) partly surrounded by local anaesthetic (hypoechoic area from 9 to 3 o´clock position relative to the nerve and indicated by the white arrow), which is sufficient for a complete nerve block.

13.8 Ulnar nerve block

13.8.1 Anatomy

The ulnar nerve is formed by parts of the medial cord and follows a superficial course (subfascial) posterior to the medial intermuscular septum, down to the sulcus of the ulnar nerve on the medial epicondyle of the humerus (Figures 13.28 and 13.29). Subsequently, the ulnar nerve passes between the two heads of the flexor carpi ulnaris muscle. At the level of the forearm, the nerve is embedded between the flexor carpi ulnaris and the superficial and profound flexor digitorum muscles (Figure 13.33). The ulnar artery joins the nerve at a variable level, between the middle and distal third of the forearm (Figure 13.34).

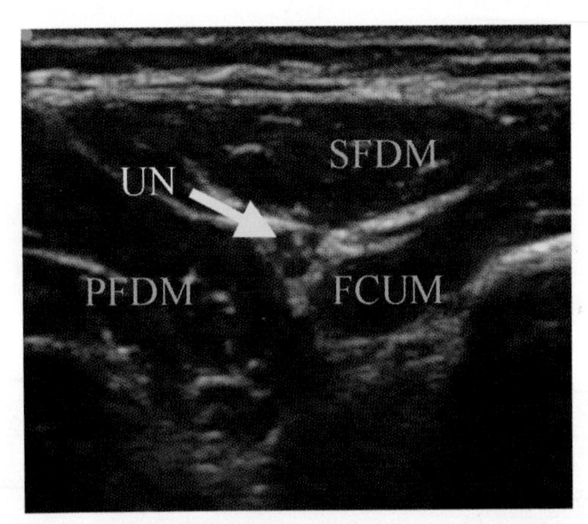

Fig. 13.33 Ultrasound image of the ulnar nerve at the level of the proximal forearm embedded between the flexor carpi ulnar muscle and the superficial and profound flexor digitorum muscles. UN: ulnar nerve; FCUM: flexor carpi ulnar muscle; SFDM: superficial flexor digitorum muscle; PFDM: profound flexor digitorum muscle; left side=radial.

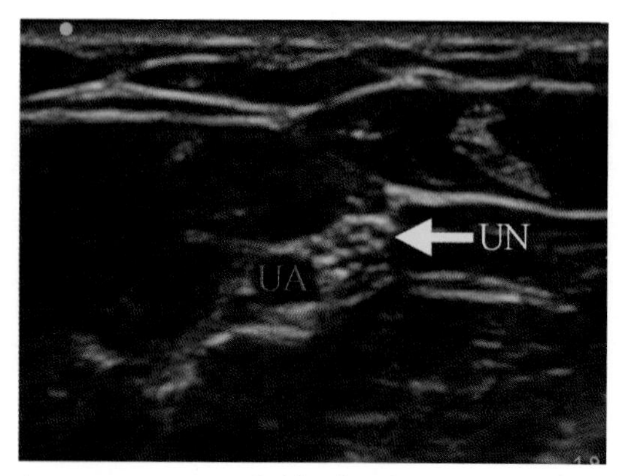

Fig. 13.34 The ulnar nerve accompanied by the ulnar artery at the level of the distal third of the forearm. UN: ulnar nerve; UA: ulnar artery; left side=radial.

13.8.2 Anatomical variations

In some cases, the ulnar nerve may run anterior to the medial epicondyle of the humerus or lie behind the condyle.

13.8.3 Ultrasound guidance technique

At the level of the forearm, the ulnar nerve appears as a hyperechoic, triangular structure (Figure 13.33) whereas above the sulcus of the ulnar nerve, it appears as a hyperechoic, oval structure (Figure 13.35).

13.8.4 Practical block technique

The ulnar nerve can be blocked above or below the level of the sulcus of the ulnar nerve. Blockade inside the sulcus should always be avoided due the risk

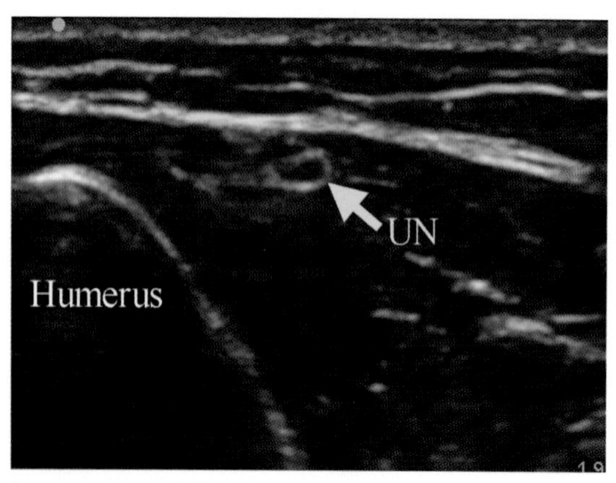

Fig. 13.35 Oval appearance of the ulnar nerve above the sulcus of the humerus. UN: ulnar nerve; left side=radial.

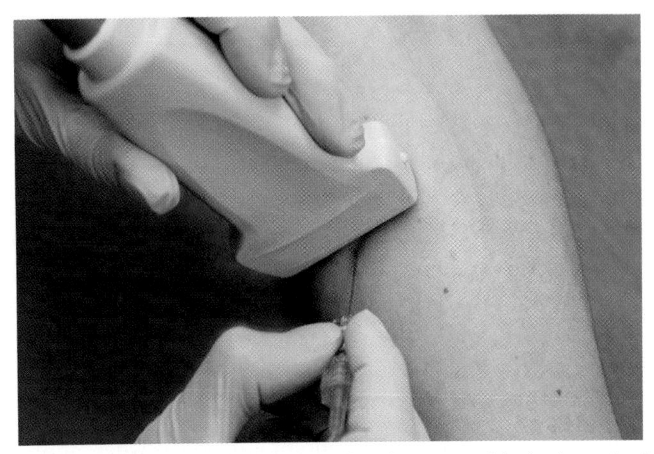

Fig. 13.36 OOP needle guidance technique for ulnar nerve blockade at the level of the proximal third of the forearm.

of puncture or pressure-related neuronal damage. The optimal position of the block is at the proximal third of the forearm where it is embedded between the flexor carpi ulnaris, the superficial flexor digitorum (humeroulnar head), and profound flexor digitorum muscles, and proximal to where the ulnar artery comes in close proximity, medial to the ulnar nerve. The preferred block technique is OOP (Figure 13.36) with the needle direction relative to the probe as illustrated for the median nerve block. To achieve a blockade with small amounts of local anaesthetic, two needle positions are required, first with the tip at the medial and then at the lateral side of the nerve.

13.8.5 **Essentials**

Block characteristic	Basic technique
Patient position	Supine, 45° abducted arm, slightly externally rotated
Ultrasound equipment	Linear probe, 25–38mm
Specific ultrasound setting	Maximum frequency
Important anatomical structures	Flexor carpi ulnaris, superficial flexor digitorum (humeroulnar head) and profound muscles
Ultrasound appearance of the neuronal structure	Hyperechoic, oval (above the sulcus of the ulnar nerve and at the distal third of the forearm) or triangular (at the proximal third of the forearm)
Expected Vienna score	1
Needle equipment	50mm, Facette tip
Technique	OOP
Estimated local anaesthetic volume	1–2mL

13.9 **Radial nerve block**

13.9.1 Anatomy

The radial nerve is formed by the posterior cord. After leaving the axilla, the nerve twists around the dorsal aspect of the humerus in a bony sulcus, accompanied by the profound brachial artery between the medial and lateral heads of the triceps muscle. In the distal third of the upper arm, the radial nerve lies between the brachialis and brachioradialis muscles. The radial nerve reaches the forearm in front of the lateral epicondyle. Here, the radial nerve is usually divided into its superficial and deep branches (Figures 13.28 and 13.29).

13.9.2 Anatomical variations

In rare cases, the radial nerve may be absent altogether, whereupon the ulnar and musculocutaneous nerves take over its area of supply. A doubled superficial branch has been observed.

13.9.3 Ultrasound guidance technique

The radial nerve can be visualized proximally to the elbow joint, between the brachialis and coracobrachialis muscles, as a hyperechoic, round or slightly oval structure (Figure 13.37). Below the elbow joint, the superficial and deep parts of the radial nerve appear as hyperechoic, round structures between the biceps tendon and brachioradialis muscle (Figure 13.38).

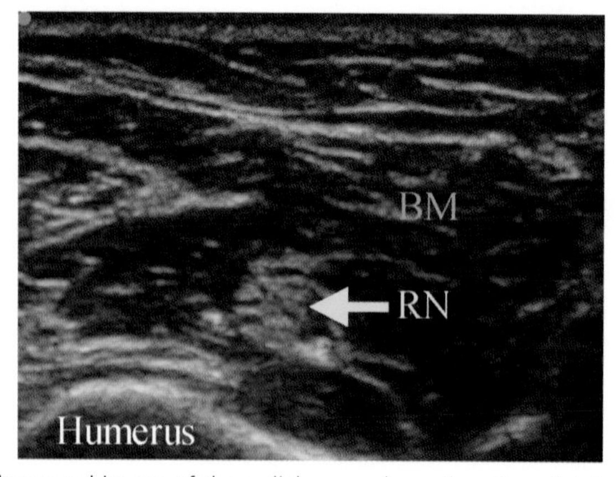

Fig. 13.37 Ultrasound image of the radial nerve above the elbow joint. RN: radial nerve; BM: brachialis muscle left side=ulnar.

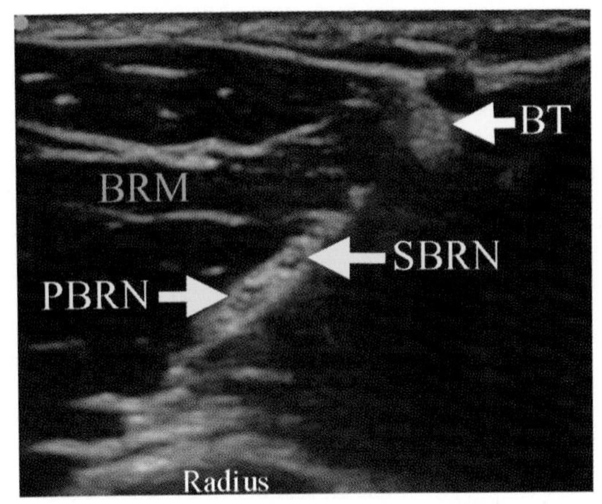

Fig. 13.38 Ultrasound image of the superficial and profound branches of the radial nerve between the brachioradialis muscle and biceps tendon. SBRN: superficial branch of the radial nerve; PBRN: profound branch of the radial nerve; BRM: brachioradialis muscle; BT: biceps tendon; left side=radial.

13.9.4 Practical block technique

Blockade of the radial nerve can be performed above or below the elbow joint. From either approach, an OOP technique is recommended with the needle positioned as illustrated in Figure 13.39. If the proximal approach is chosen, a two-injection technique with a needle tip position at the medial and lateral side of the nerve guarantees optimal success. In cases where the more distal

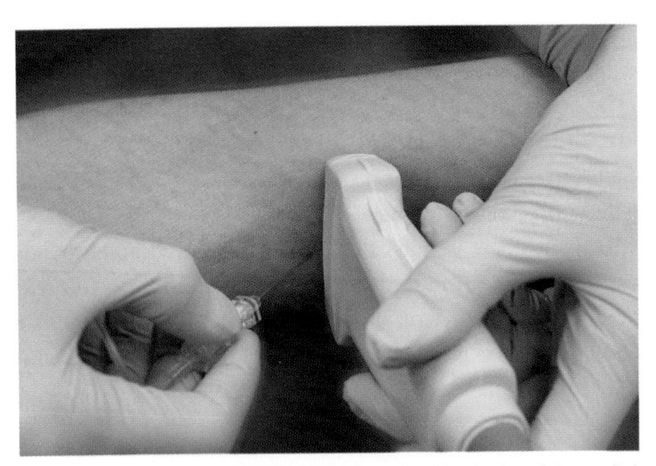

Fig. 13.39 OOP plane needle guidance technique for blockade of the radial nerve above the elbow joint; right side=proximal.

approach is performed, a single-injection technique with a needle tip position between the superficial and profound part of the nerve usually provides a sufficient spread of local anaesthetic around the nerve structures.

13.9.5 **Essentials**

Block characteristic	Basic technique
Patient position	Supine, arm slightly abducted
Ultrasound equipment	Linear probe, 25–38mm
Specific ultrasound setting	Maximum frequency
Important anatomical structures	Brachial muscle (above the elbow), brachioradialis muscle, and biceps tendon (below the elbow)
Ultrasound appearance of the neuronal structures	Above the elbow joint: hyperechoic, round to slightly oval. Below the elbow joint: always divided into its superficial and deep parts, both branches hyperechoic, round
Expected Vienna score	1–2
Needle equipment	50mm, Facette tip
Technique	OOP
Estimated local anaesthetic volume	2–3mL

13.10 **Implications of upper limb blocks in children**

Upper limb blocks in children are of major importance due to the large number of cases and indications. In principle, all techniques are possible as described in adults. The *supraclavicular approach* seems to be the most practicable technique. The entire neuronal structures of the brachial plexus are in close proximity to each other and easily accessible. In cases of fractures of the upper extremity, the supraclavicular approach can be performed in a neutral position and therefore, painful abduction of the upper extremity can be avoided.

The axillary approach in children under 3 years old may be technically difficult because of the extreme superficial position of the target structures. Thus, even when an axillary brachial plexus block is indicated in children under 3, a supraclavicular approach should be considered.

The algorithm for an appropriate management of upper limb fractures in children is explained in Chapter 7.

Suggested further reading

Chan, V., Perlas, A., Rawson, R., Odukoya, O., (2003). Ultrasound-guided supraclavicular brachial plexus block. *Anesthesia & Analgesia*, 97(5), pp.1514–7.

Greher, M., Retzl, G., Niel, P., Kamholz, L., Marhofer, P., Kapral, S., (2002). Ultrasonographic assessment of topographic anatomy in volunteers suggests a modification of the infraclavicular vertical brachial plexus block. *British Journal of Anaesthesia*, 88(5), pp.632–6.

Kapral, S., Greher, M., Huber, G., Willschke, H., Kettner, S., Kdolsky, R., Marhofer, P., (2008). Ultrasonographic guidance improves the success rate of interscalene plexus blockade. *Regional Anesthesia and Pain Medicine*, 33(3), pp.253–8.

Marhofer, P., Sitzwohl, C., Greher, M., Kapral, S., (2004). Ultrasound guidance for infraclavicular brachial plexus anaesthesia in children. *Anaesthesia*, 59(7), pp.642–6.

Marhofer, P., Willschke, H., Kettner, S., (2006). Imaging techniques for regional nerve blockade and vascular cannulation in children. *Current Opinion in Anesthesiology*, 19(3), pp.293–300.

McCartney, C., Xu, D., Constantinescu, C., Abbas, S., Chan, V., (2007). Ultrasound examination of peripheral nerves in the forearm. *Regional Anesthesia and Pain Medicine*, 32(5), pp.434–9.

Retzl, G., Kapral, S., Greher, M., Mauritz, W., (2001). Ultrasonographic findings of the axillary part of the brachial plexus. *Anesthesia & Analgesia*, 92(5), pp.1271–5.

Sauter, A., Smith, H., Stubhaug, A., Dodgson, M., Klaastad, Ø., (2006). Use of magnetic resonance imaging to define the anatomical location closest to all three cords of the infraclavicular brachial plexus. *Anesthesia & Analgesia*, 103(6), pp.1574–6.

Chapter 14

Lower extremity blocks

14.1 General anatomical considerations

The *lumbar plexus* derives from the ventral rami of the spinal nerves L1–L3 and parts of L4 (furcal nerve). The first lumbar ramus commonly receives a branch from T12. The lumbar plexus is formed within the posterior portion of the psoas major muscle. The branches of the lumbar plexus are the iliohypogastric, ilioinguinal, genitofemoral, femoral, lateral femoral cutaneous, and obturator nerves.

The *sacral plexus* is formed by parts of the ventral rami L4 and L5 (lumbosacral trunk) together with the ventral rami of the sacral nerves S1–S3. The sacral plexus is located within the pelvis on the ventral surface of the piriformis muscle. The major branches relevant for regional anaesthesia are the sciatic and posterior femoral cutaneous nerves. Due to its location within the pelvis, the sacral plexus cannot be accessed with today's ultrasound skills.

14.2 Psoas compartment block

14.2.1 Anatomy (Figure 14.1)

The term 'psoas compartment block' was introduced decades ago to describe a potential space between the psoas major and quadratus lumborum muscles. However, several anatomical studies have since demonstrated that the lumbar plexus is located within the substance of the psoas major muscle. Therefore, the term 'psoas compartment' should be used to describe the layer within the muscle which contains the lumbar plexus and its branches. The iliohypogastric and ilioinguinal nerves emerge from the upper lateral border of the psoas muscle whereas the genitofemoral nerve leaves the muscle on its ventral surface. The femoral nerve exits the muscle on its posterolateral surface to lay in the gutter between the psoas major and iliacus muscles. The lateral femoral cutaneous nerve emerges from the lateral border of the psoas muscle. In contrast, the obturator nerve descends within the muscle and emerges from its posteromedial border. At the level L4–5, the main nerves of the lumbar plexus (femoral, obturator, and lateral femoral cutaneous) are situated within the posterior part of the psoas major muscle in the vast majority of patients. Here, they can be accessed by a posterior approach.

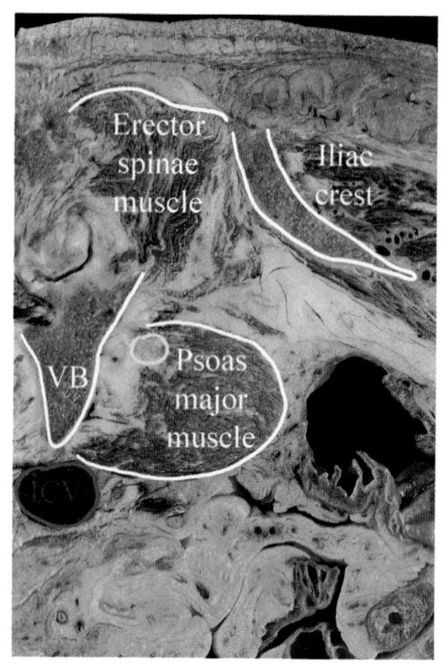

Fig. 14.1 Cross-sectional anatomical image of the lumbar paravertebral region. The yellow circle indicates the L1 nerve root inside the psoas major muscle. ICV: inferior cava vein; VB: vertebral body; left side=medial.

14.2.2 Anatomical variations

The lumbar plexus may be also encountered in high (prefixed) or low (postfixed) form. In the prefixed form, the plexus receives a branch from T12 whereas in the postfixed form, the ventral ramus L5 contributes to the plexus. In rare cases, the entire plexus is located posterior to the psoas major muscle, adjacent to the lumbar transverse processes. This variant should be considered when nerve stimulation fails to locate the plexus within the psoas muscle. Additionally, the femoral nerve shows a remarkable degree of branching within the psoas muscle in some cases. Two or three branches of the femoral nerve may be found within the psoas major muscle. This might explain partial block effects since the respective branches are separated by more or less muscular tissue.

14.2.3 Ultrasound guidance technique

Ultrasonography of the lumbar paravertebral region provides reliable and detailed imaging of the psoas major muscle and the surrounding structures. Curved array transducers operating at lower frequencies have been found to be the best choice for this purpose. Due to the deep location of the lumbar plexus and the typical echo texture of the psoas major muscle, the delineation of neural structures is difficult in the adult population since the distance between the skin and the plexus increases with body mass index. Thus, we recommend the additional use of nerve stimulation to help locate the lumbar plexus.

Patient positioning is equivalent to the classic technique: lateral decubitus position with the operated side uppermost, hips and knees slightly flexed. Identifying the lumbar levels can be best achieved by means of a longitudinal paravertebral sonogram showing the lumbar transverse processes. They can be counted in a cephalic direction, beginning at the posterior surface of the sacrum. The L4/L5 transverse processes, and subsequently the intertransverse space, should be identified. The transducer should then be rotated into a transverse plane to delineate the psoas major muscle at the intertransverse space. Best imaging of the entire paravertebral region is achieved with a transducer position 5–6cm lateral from the spinous processes. Here, the muscle has an oval-shaped configuration with an echo texture typically consisting of hyperechoic striations on a hypoechoic background. The hyperechoic structures correspond to tendon-like bundles of fibrous tissue within the muscle that can be misinterpreted as neural structures.

The adjacent structures are the lower pole of the respective kidney laterally (may descend down to L4, especially during deep inspiration), the adjacent vertebral body medially, the erector spinae muscle dorsally, and the retroperitoneal

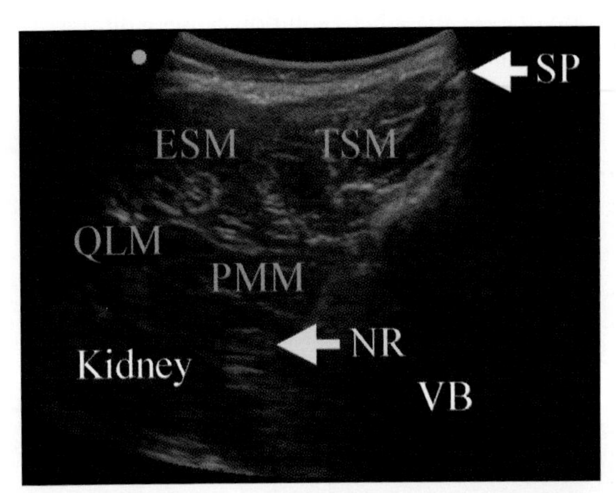

Fig. 14.2 Ultrasound illustration of the lumbar paravertebral region at the L3/4 level. The position of the nerve root can be estimated between the posterior and middle third in cases when the nerve structures are not directly visible. NR: nerve root; PMM: psoas major muscle; QLM: quadratus lumborum muscle; TSM: transversospinal muscle; ESM: erector spinae muscle; SP: spinous process; VB: vertebral body; left side=lateral.

space ventrally. The quadratus lumborum muscle is situated posterolateral to the psoas major muscle (Figure 14.2).

14.2.4 Practical block technique

After identifying the relevant structures at the L4–5 level, both a cutaneous and a deep subcutaneous infiltration should be performed close to the medial side of the transducer. A 100–150mm long needle is inserted using the IP technique (Figure 14.3). The needle is gently advanced through the erector spinae to access the posterior part of the psoas major muscle. Recent evolution in needle technology may facilitate an improved visibility of the body of the needle during this technique. Piercing the inner layer of the thoracolumbal fascia can be felt as a clear pop and occasionally provokes a painful sensation.

In most cases, the lumbar plexus is located within the posterior and middle thirds of the psoas major muscle. Using a nerve stimulator, twitches of the quadriceps muscle are commonly obtained at a depth of 6–9cm, depending on the body mass index. A stimulation threshold of 0.4–0.5mA is satisfactory. Twitches of the adductor muscles indicate a medial needle position that should be corrected as an epidural spread of local anaesthetic is possible. Although the correct needle position should be confirmed by ultrasound imaging, an initial test dose can be recommended to rule out an intrathecal spread in cases of uncertainty. After careful aspiration, the local anaesthetic solution should be injected in fractions to detect acute systemic toxicity, since false-negative aspiration tests are possible. Injection of local anaesthetic solution causes a diffuse distension of the psoas major muscle in contrast to superficial blocks where a distinct volume

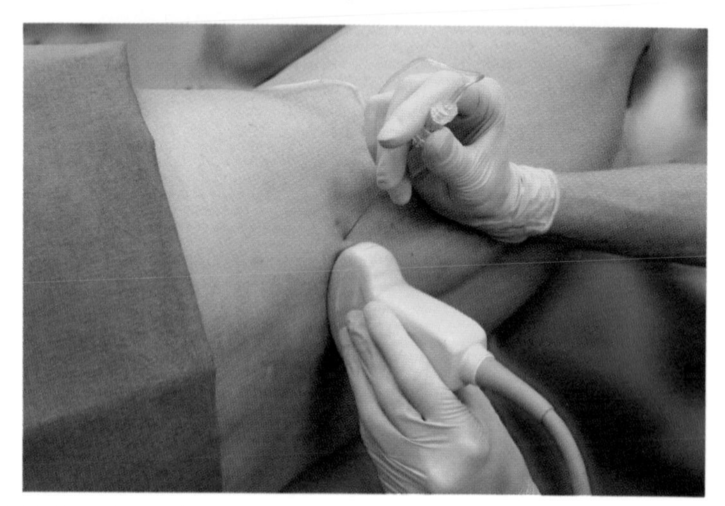

Fig. 14.3 IP needle guidance technique for the psoas compartment block with a needle position from lateral.

effect is recognized. A total volume of 25mL of local anaesthetic solution usually provides a sufficient block of the main branches of the lumbar plexus.

14.2.5 Essentials

Block characteristic	Advanced technique
Patient position	Lateral decubitus position with the operated side uppermost, hips and knees slightly flexed
Ultrasound equipment	Curved array probe
Specific ultrasound setting	Low frequency, choose 'abdominal' preset
Important anatomical structures	Psoas major, quadratus lumborum and erector spinae muscles, vertebral body, lower pole of the kidney
Ultrasound appearance of the neuronal structures	–
Expected Vienna score	4
Needle equipment	80–150mm, Facette tip
Technique	IP
Estimated local anaesthetic volume	20–25mL

14.3 Femoral nerve block

14.3.1 Anatomy

The femoral nerve as the largest branch of the lumbar plexus arises from the ventral rami L1–4. It passes distally between the psoas major and iliacus muscles to reach the lacuna musculorum. At this site, the femoral nerve is located beneath the inguinal ligament, lateral to the femoral vessels and on the anterior surface of the iliopsoas muscle covered by its fascia. Subsequently, the nerve divides into several branches: an anterior group for sensory supply, and a medial and lateral group for motor supply (Figure 14.4).

14.3.2 Anatomical variations

The femoral nerve may arise from T12–L4 (prefixed plexus) or L1–5 (postfixed plexus). Instead of running on the anterior surface of the iliopsoas muscle, the nerve may pierce the latter. The nerve has also been found between the femoral vessels.

14.3.3 Ultrasound guidance technique

Using a high-frequency linear probe, the nerve should be located above or slightly distal to the inguinal ligament. The nerve is located in a very close

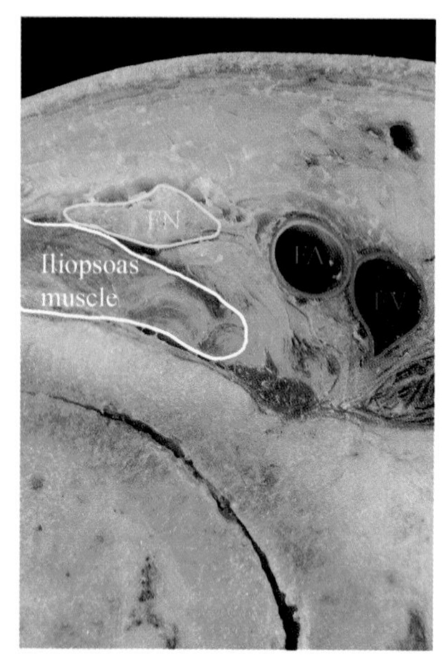

Fig. 14.4 Cross-sectional anatomical image of the femoral nerve lateral to the inguinal vessels. FN: femoral nerve; FA: femoral artery; FV: femoral vein; left side=lateral.

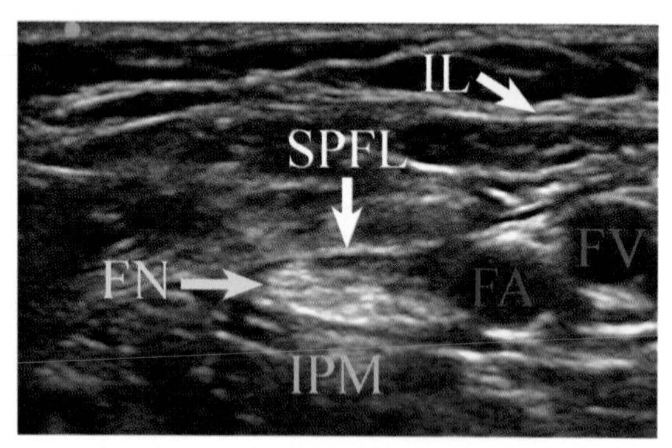

Fig. 14.5 Ultrasound illustration of the femoral nerve with a probe position as shown in Figure 14.6. The nerve is below the superficial part of the fascia lata and the inguinal ligament and lateral to the femoral artery and femoral vein. The iliopsoas muscle is beneath the nerve. FN: femoral nerve; SPFL: superficial part of the fascia lata; IL: inguinal ligament; FA: femoral artery; FV: femoral vein; IPM: iliopsoas muscle; left side=lateral.

position relative to the psoas major muscle and the femoral artery (Figure 14.5) and may appear less echoic on ultrasonography than other nerves. The superficial portion of the fascia lata can be identified above the nerve and the femoral vessels. The iliopectineal fascia divides the lacuna musculorum from the vessels and ultrasound identification is usually possible after the administration of local anaesthetic. Orientation of the probe in a cranial direction may improve the visibility of the nerve due to its anisotropy.

14.3.4 Practical block technique

Since the femoral nerve divides slightly distal to the inguinal ligament in several branches, blockade should be performed as proximally as possible, but always below the inguinal ligament. As described above, the decreased echogenicity of the femoral nerve may make it difficult to visualize. Therefore, careful probe adjustments should be performed to optimize the visibility of the nerve. The large femoral vessels serve as clear guidance structures. The OOP needle direction is the preferred technique for this block (Figure 14.6). Because the nerve is embedded in muscle structures, the local anaesthetic should be administered carefully in order to avoid intraneuronal injection.

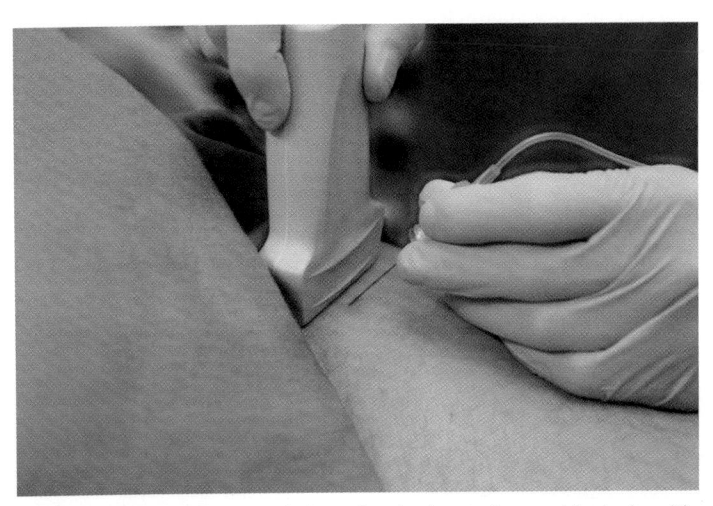

Fig. 14.6 OOP needle guidance technique for the femoral nerve blockade with a needle position from caudal.

14.3.5 Essentials

Block characteristic	Basic technique
Patient position	Supine, slightly externally rotated lower extremity
Ultrasound equipment	Linear probe, 38mm
Specific ultrasound setting	Maximum frequency
Important anatomical structures	Femoral artery, superficial portion of the fascia lata, iliopsoas muscle
Ultrasound appearance of the neuronal structures	Impaired echogenicity, round to oval
Expected Vienna score	2–3
Needle equipment	50mm, Facette tip
Technique	OOP
Estimated local anaesthetic volume	5mL

14.4 Saphenous nerve block

14.4.1 Anatomy

The saphenous nerve is a pure sensory branch of the femoral nerve. It lies inside the adductor canal in front of the femoral artery down to the lower part of the adductor magnus muscle, where the nerve separates from the artery to descend vertically to the medial side of the knee behind the sartorius muscle. After piercing the fascia lata, the nerve lies between the tendons of the gracilis and sartorius muscles and becomes subcutaneous. *Infrapatellar branches* of the saphenous nerve supply a skin area distal to the patella. At the tibial side of the leg, the saphenous nerve is accompanied by the great saphenous vein (Figures 14.7 and 14.8).

14.4.2 Anatomical variations

In some cases, the saphenous nerve may pierce the sartorius muscle. It has also been found to terminate at the level of the knee joint. A branch of the tibial nerve may then cover its area of supply. The infrapatellar branch may originate from the branch to the vastus medialis muscle and may pierce, pass superficially, or pass beneath the sartorius muscle.

14.4.3 Ultrasound guidance technique

The femoral artery is visualized on the medial side of the thigh. Where the artery is situated deeply, colour Doppler scanning might be useful. The saphenous nerve is located above the artery and appears as a hyperechoic, round

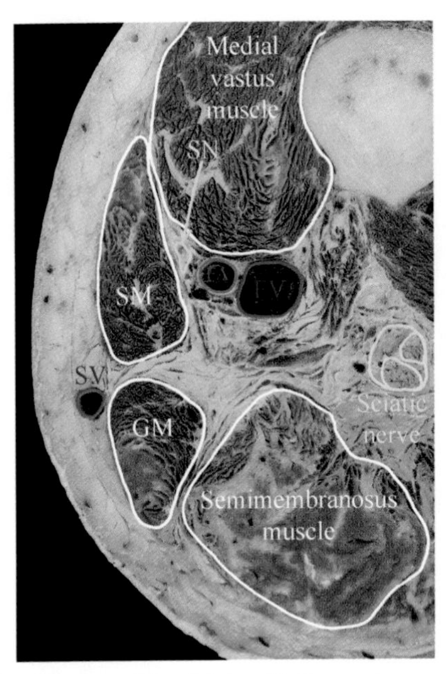

Fig. 14.7 Cross-sectional image of the thigh with the saphenous nerve adjacent to the femoral artery. The sciatic nerve appears lateral to the semimembranosus muscle. SN: saphenous nerve; FA: femoral artery; FV: femoral vein; SV: saphenous vein; GM: gracilis muscle; SM: sartorius muscle; left side=medial.

structure (Figure 14.9). Tracking the nerve and artery in a distal direction shows that the femoral artery descends down the adductor canal whereas the nerve moves in a more superficial position behind the sartorius muscle (Figure 14.10).

14.4.4 Practical block technique

Once the saphenous nerve is identified behind the sartorius muscle as a hyperechoic, round structure, the block can be performed using the IP technique (Figure 14.11). The needle should be guided carefully behind the sartorius muscle until the nerve is approached.

More distal and anterior to the medial malleolus, the nerve can be blocked using the OOP technique. The probe should be placed with minimal pressure in order to avoid compression of the great saphenous vein which carries the risk of inadvertently and unknowingly positioning the needle tip intravascularly. We prefer the proximal blockade of the saphenous nerve due to a better visualization and a larger spectrum of indications for this block (e.g. knee surgery).

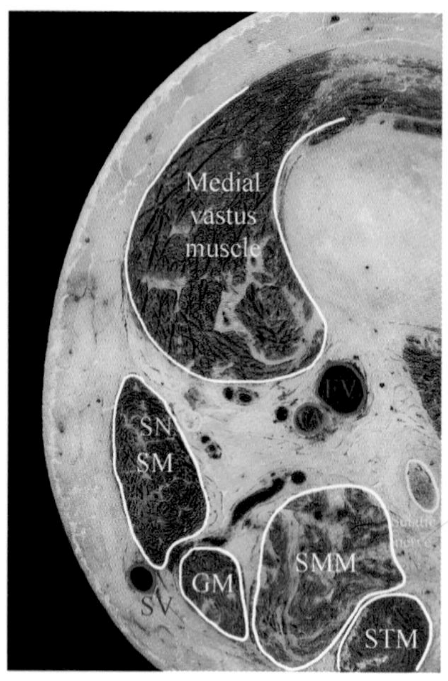

Fig. 14.8 Cross-sectional image of the thigh with the saphenous nerve behind the sartorius muscle and the femoral vessels already inside the adductor canal. The sciatic nerve is in a position lateral to the semimembranosus muscle. SN: saphenous nerve; SM: sartorius muscle; FA: femoral artery, FV: femoral vein; SMM: semimembranosus muscle; GM: gracilis muscle; STM: semitendinosus muscle; SV: saphenous vein; left side=medial.

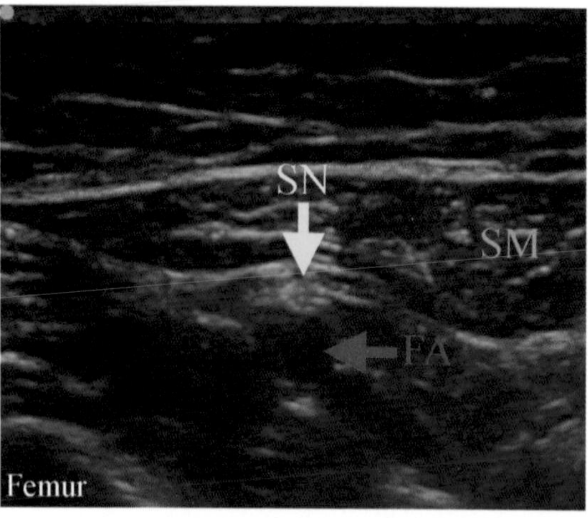

Fig. 14.9 Ultrasound appearance of the saphenous nerve in a 12 o´clock position relative to the femoral artery. SN: saphenous nerve; FA: femoral artery; SM: sartorius muscle; left side=caudal.

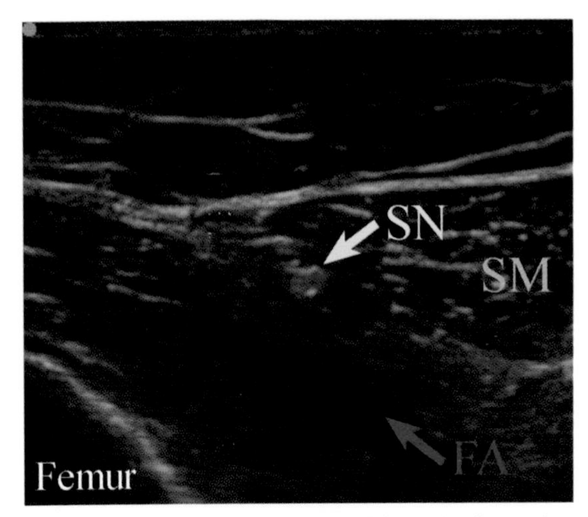

Fig. 14.10 The saphenous nerve already separated from the femoral artery (impaired visibility due to its deep position). SN: saphenous nerve; FA: femoral artery; SM: sartorius muscle; left side=caudal.

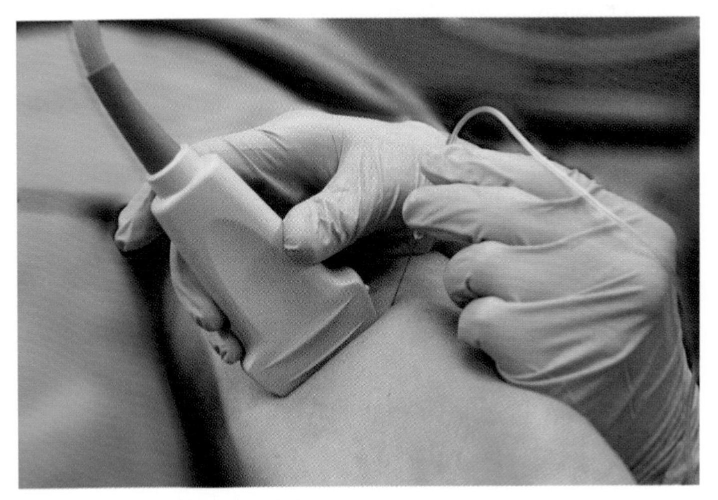

Fig. 14.11 IP needle guidance technique for saphenous nerve blockade.

14.4.5 **Essentials**

Block characteristic	Basic technique
Patient position	Supine, slightly externally rotated lower leg and slightly flexed knee
Ultrasound equipment	38mm, linear probe
Specific ultrasound setting	Medium frequency when the femoral artery in visualized, high frequency during tracking of the saphenous nerve
Important anatomical structures	Femoral artery, sartorius muscle
Ultrasound appearance of the neuronal structures	Hyperechoic, round
Expected Vienna score	1–2
Needle equipment	50mm, Facette tip
Technique	Proximal: IP Distal: OOP
Estimated local anaesthetic volume	Proximal: 2–3mL Distal: 1–2mL

14.4.6 **Blockade of the infrapatellar branch**

14.4.6.1 Anatomy

At the level of the knee, the saphenous nerve gives off a large infrapatellar branch which pierces the sartorius muscle and the fascia lata to supply the skin in front of the patella. The infrapatellar branch later forms the plexus patellae, together with branches of the lateral cutaneous femoral nerve.

14.4.6.2 Ultrasound guidance technique

Once the saphenous nerve is detected below the sartorius muscle, the infrapatellar branch can be visualized as a hyperechoic, round structure located more superficially below the sartorius muscle compared with the saphenous nerve (Figure 14.12). On tracking the branch more distally, it is possible to detect piercing of the sartorius muscle.

14.4.6.3 Practical block technique

The infrapatellar branch can be blocked slightly distally to the described site of blockade for the saphenous nerve using an IP technique. The technique itself is exactly the same as described for the saphenous nerve (see Section 14.4).

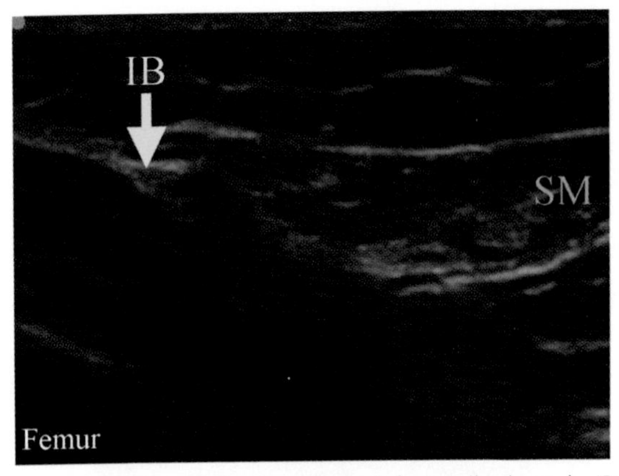

Fig. 14.12 Ultrasonographic appearance of one infrapatellar branch. IB: infrapatellar branch; SM: sartorius muscle; left side=caudal.

14.4.6.4 Essentials

Block characteristic	Basic technique
Patient position	Supine, slightly externally rotated lower leg and slightly flexed knee
Ultrasound equipment	38mm, linear probe
Specific ultrasound setting	High frequency
Important anatomical structures	Saphenous nerve, sartorius muscle
Ultrasound appearance of the neuronal structures	Round, hyperechoic
Expected Vienna score	2
Needle equipment	50mm, Facette tip
Technique	IP
Estimated local anaesthetic volume	2mL

14.5 **Lateral femoral cutaneous nerve block**

14.5.1 Anatomy

The lateral femoral cutaneous nerve usually arises from the ventral rami L2–3. It crosses the iliacus muscle obliquely toward the anterior superior iliac spine, where it passes medially to the latter below the inguinal ligament, over the sartorius muscle and into the thigh (Figure 14.13).

14.5.2 Anatomical variations

The lateral femoral cutaneous nerve may arise from L1–2 (prefixed plexus) or from L3–4 (postfixed plexus). It may be missing on one side and be replaced

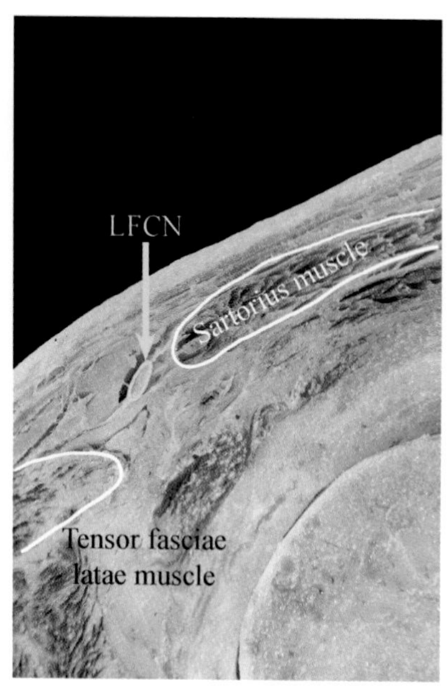

Fig. 14.13 Anatomical cross-sectional view of the lateral inguinal area with the lateral femoral cutaneous nerve lateral to the sartorius muscle. LFCN: lateral femoral cutaneous nerve; left side=lateral.

by an anterior cutaneous branch of the femoral nerve or by the ilioinguinal nerve. The nerve may pass beneath the inguinal ligament more medially (between the anterior superior iliac spine and the femoral vessels). It may pierce, pass anteriorly to, or pass posteriorly to the sartorius muscle.

14.5.3 Ultrasound guidance technique

The lateral femoral cutaneous nerve is in a position closely medial to the anterior superior iliac spine, and anterior, within, or posterior to the sartorius muscle. Since the sartorius muscle originates from the anterior superior iliac spine, the hyperechoic appearance of the origin of the latter impairs the visibility of the nerve. Improved visibility may be achieved with a more distal position of the probe. The nerve itself should appear as a hyperechoic, round structure anterior to the belly of the sartorius muscle or in the triangular space between the sartorius and tensor fasciae latae muscles (Figure 14.14).

14.5.4 Practical block technique

Following the administration of larger volumes of local anaesthetics (20mL) during femoral nerve blockade, an additional block of the lateral cutaneous femoral nerve can be achieved. When a single blockade of the lateral cutaneous

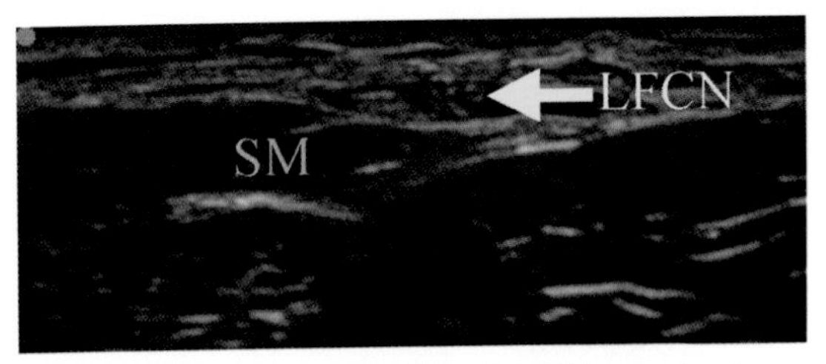

Fig. 14.14 Ultrasonographic appearance of the lateral femoral cutaneous nerve slightly medial the anterior superior iliac spine (right to the nerve). LFCN: lateral femoral cutaneous nerve; SM: sartorius muscle; left side=medial.

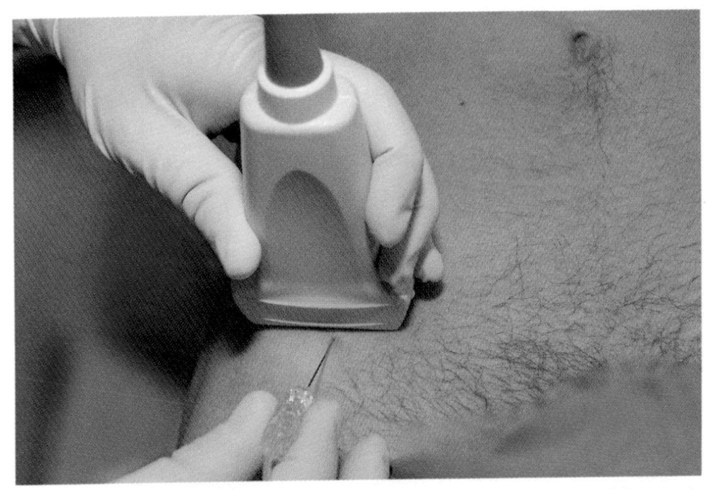

Fig. 14.15 OOP needle guidance technique for blockade of the lateral femoral cutaneous nerve medial the anterior superior iliac spine.

femoral nerve is indicated, the nerve should be visualized medially and slightly caudally to the anterior superior iliac spine, above the belly of the sartorius muscle, using the OOP technique with a needle position below the probe (Figure 14.15).

14.5.5 **Essentials**

Block characteristic	Basic technique
Patient position	Supine
Ultrasound equipment	38mm, linear probe
Specific ultrasound setting	High frequency
Important anatomical structures	Anterior superior iliac spine, sartorius muscle, inguinal ligament

Ultrasound appearance of the neuronal structures	Hyperechoic, round
Expected Vienna score	2
Needle equipment	50mm, Facette tip
Technique	OOP
Estimated local anaesthetic volume	1–2mL

14.6 **Obturator nerve block**

14.6.1 **Anatomy** (Figure 14.16)

The obturator nerve commonly arises from the ventral divisions of L2–4. It emerges through the upper and lateral part of the obturator foramen, down to the medial side of the thigh (together with the obturator artery in the obturator canal), and divides into an anterior (between the adductor longus and adductor brevis muscles) and a posterior branch (between the adductor brevis and adductor magnus muscles).

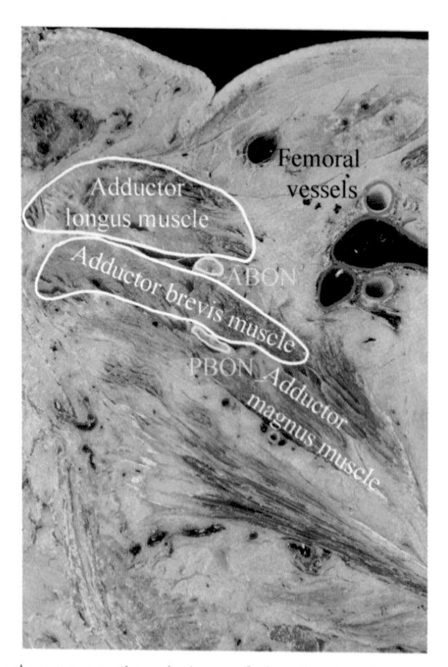

Fig. 14.16 Anatomical cross-sectional view of the thigh with the anterior and posterior branches of the obturator nerve between the adductor muscles. ABON: anterior branch of the obturator nerve; PBON: posterior branch of the obturator nerve; left side=lateral.

14.6.2 Anatomical variations

The obturator nerve may arise from the ventral rami L1–4 (prefixed plexus) or L2–5 (postfixed plexus). Both branches of the nerve have been found to pass posteriorly to the adductor brevis muscle. An accessory obturator nerve may be encountered arising most commonly from L3–4 (also L2–4, L2–3, or L3). It usually runs together with the obturator nerve, but descends along the psoas major muscle to cross the anterior brim of the pelvis. The accessory obturator nerve passes beneath the pectineus muscle to terminate in three branches. These branches supply the adductor muscles and the hip joint in a variable manner.

14.6.3 Ultrasound guidance technique

The probe should be carefully moved from its position above the greater femoral vessels in a medial direction until the pectineus, long adductor, and short adductor muscles are visualized. The anterior branch of the obturator nerve is located inside this typical 'muscular triangle' (Figure 14.17). Visualization of this nerve can sometimes be improved by injection of local anaesthetic solution. The posterior branch is located between the adductor brevis and magnus muscles.

14.6.4 Practical block technique

Both nerves should be approached by means of the IP technique and the needle inserted laterally to the probe (Figure 14.18). Advancement of the needle between the pectineus and long adductor muscle (Figure 14.19) avoids unnecessary tissue damage.

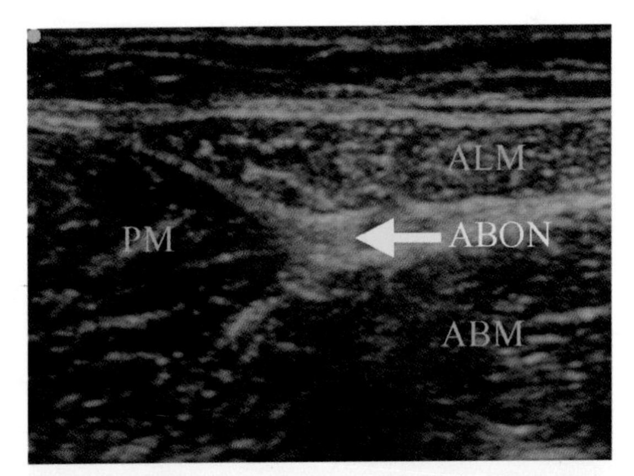

Fig. 14.17 Ultrasound image of the anterior branch of the obturator nerve between the pectineus, long adductor, and short adductor muscles on the medial side of the thigh. ABON: anterior branch obturator nerve; PM: pectineus muscle; ALM: adductor longus muscle; ABM: adductor brevis muscle; left side=lateral.

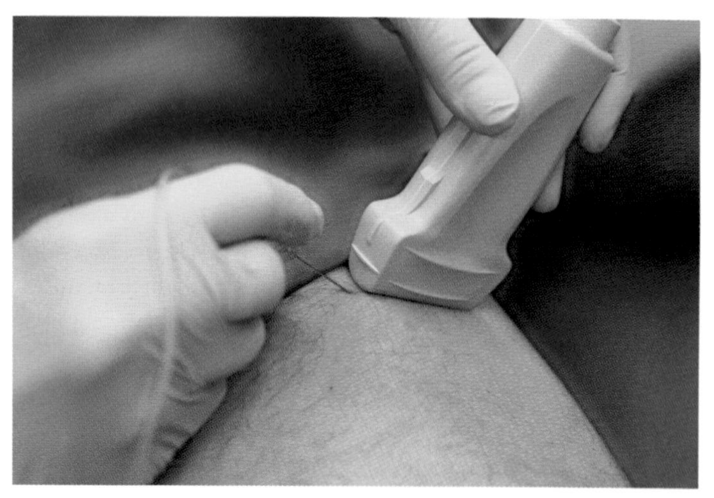

Fig. 14.18 IP needle guidance technique for blockade of the two branches of the obturator nerve with a lateral–medial needle direction.

14.6.5 Essentials

Block characteristic	Intermediate technique
Patient position	Supine, externally rotated leg
Ultrasound equipment	38mm, linear probe
Specific ultrasound setting	High frequency
Important anatomical structures	Pectineus, adductor longus, brevis and magnus modes
Ultrasound appearance of the neuronal structures	Hyperechoic, round
Expected Vienna score	2–3
Needle equipment	50 or 70mm, Facette tip
Technique	IP
Estimated local anaesthetic volume	3–4mL each

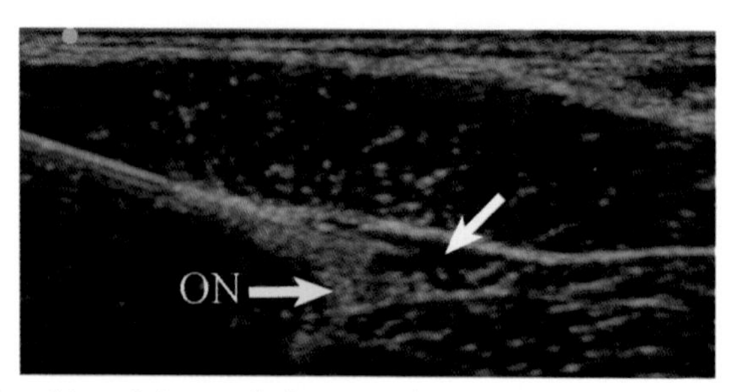

Fig. 14.19 IP position of the needle between the pectineus and long adductor muscles for blockade of the obturator nerve. The white arrow indicates the local anaesthetic solution. ON: obturator nerve; left side=lateral.

14.7 **Sciatic nerve blocks**

Various approaches to the sciatic nerve are applicable using ultrasonographic-guided techniques. In the following chapter, we discuss five approaches from proximal to distal until the sciatic nerve divides into the common peroneal and tibial nerves. Despite the fact that the sciatic nerve is the largest nerve in the human body, ultrasonographic visualization is sometimes difficult. This might be due to the lack of easy identifiable landmarks such as large vessels and the remarkable anisotropic behaviour. Therefore, careful probe adjustment and profound anatomical knowledge are necessary for a reliable identification of the sciatic nerve at all levels.

14.7.1 Transgluteal approach

14.7.1.1 Anatomy

The sciatic nerve usually arises from the ventral rami L4–S3. Once the sciatic nerve passes out of the pelvis through the infrapiriformic foramen, it is located between the piriformis, greater gluteus, gemelli, and quadratus femoris muscles. The sciatic nerve is accompanied medially by the posterior femoral cutaneous nerve. Since several branches supply the hip joint, this approach should be used as part of a regional anaesthesia concept for hip surgery.

14.7.1.2 Anatomical variations

In most cases, the sciatic nerve passes beneath the piriformis muscle. In a few cases, the nerve may pierce the piriformis muscle (most frequently only the peroneal part) or pass above it. The level of division into the common peroneal and tibial nerves may be encountered at any level between its origin, the lower thigh.

14.7.1.3 Ultrasound guidance technique

Due to the deep location of the nerve, a sector probe should be used. The optimal position of the patient is lateral with a slightly flexed hip and knee. The probe should be placed in a connecting line between the coccygeus and greater trochanter. The sciatic nerve can be expected at a depth between 5 and 8cm as a hyperechoic, flat to round structure (Figure 14.20). Because of the fact that medium to low frequencies are used in this approach, the internal structure of the nerve cannot be visualized as compared with more superficial nerves. The cutaneous femoris posterior nerve in that position is constantly medial to the sciatic nerve and direct visualization may be difficult due to the smaller diameter of the nerve.

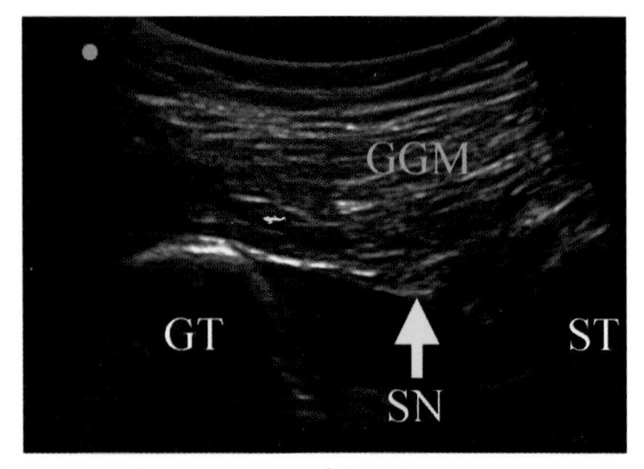

Fig. 14.20 Ultrasonographic appearance of the sciatic nerve between the greater trochanter and the sciatic tuber at the infragluteal level. SN: sciatic nerve; GT: greater trochanter; ST: sciatic tuber; GGM: greater gluteus muscle; left side=lateral.

14.7.1.4 Practical block technique

Once the sciatic nerve is adequately visualized, the block can be performed using an IP or OOP technique (Figure 14.21). At least two needle positions are necessary for a successful blockade, one lateral and one medial. It is important to note that the onset times for proximal sciatic nerve blocks are long.

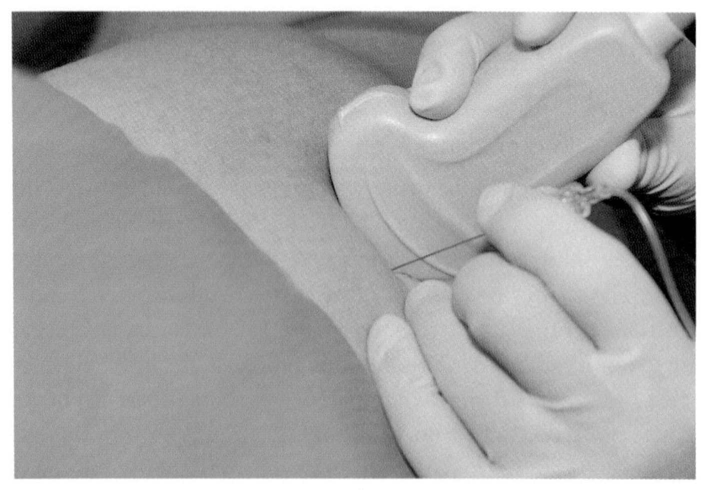

Fig. 14.21 OOP needle guidance technique for the transgluteal sciatic nerve blockade.

14.7.1.5 Essentials

Block characteristic	Intermediate technique
Patient position	Lateral, hip and knee slightly flexed
Ultrasound equipment	Sector probe
Specific ultrasound setting	Middle to low frequency
Important anatomical structures	Greater gluteus, gemelli and quadratus femoris muscles
Ultrasound appearance of the neuronal structures	Hyperechoic, round to oval
Expected Vienna score	3
Needle equipment	80–120mm, Facette tip
Technique	OOP or IP
Estimated local anaesthetic volume	12–16mL

14.7.2 Anterior approach

14.7.2.1 Anatomy

See other proximal approaches to the sciatic nerve.

14.7.2.2 Ultrasound guidance technique

Using the anterior technique to block the sciatic nerve, it lies between the minor trochanter and the sciatic tuber. The anterior technique for blockade of the sciatic nerve is relatively comfortable for the patient from the positioning point of view (supine). Nevertheless, the sciatic nerve is in its deepest position using the anterior technique. Once the minor trochanter and sciatic tuber are visualized, the nerve lies between these bone structures and below the rectus femoris and greater adductor muscles (Figure 14.22). A low frequency sector probe should be used to visualize the nerve as a hyperechoic, oval to round structure.

14.7.2.3 Practical block technique

Once the nerve is visualized between the minor trochanter and sciatic tuber, the blockade should be performed between the rectus femoris and sartorius muscles using the IP technique with a needle position in an absolute perpendicular direction from the medial side (Figure 14.23). The length of the needle depends on the initial measurement of the depth of the nerve. Usually 8 to 12cm needles are adequate. The needle should be placed medially

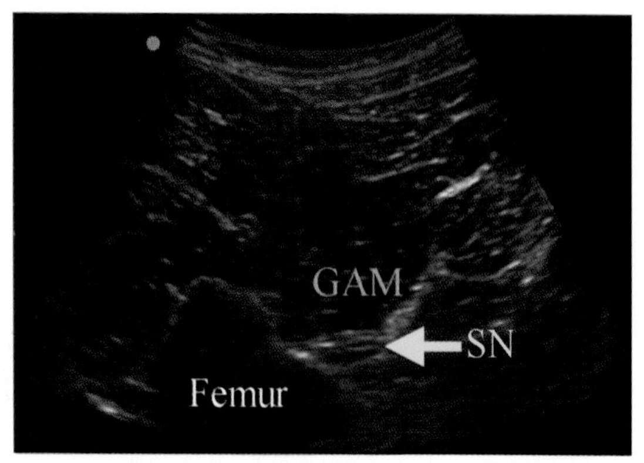

Fig. 14.22 Ultrasonographic appearance of the sciatic nerve medial to and below the femur by performing the anterior approach. SN: sciatic nerve; GAM: greater adductor muscle; left side=lateral.

and laterally the nerve and care should be taken to avoid puncture of the femoral vessels (Figure 14.24). Prior to the administration of local anaesthetic, careful aspiration is necessary since small vessels are difficult to visualize in that depth.

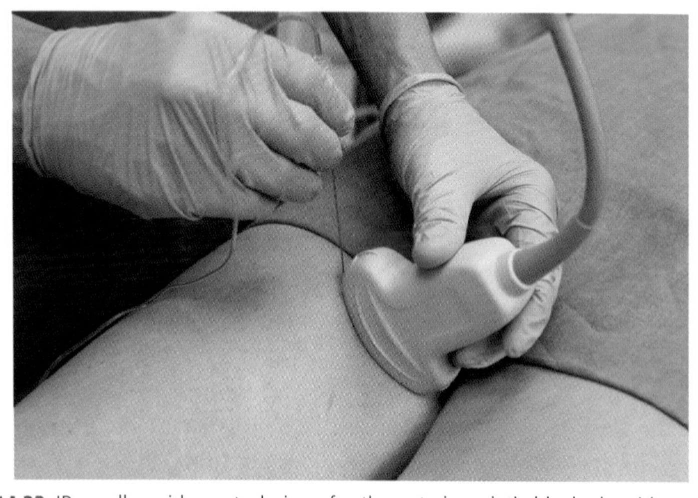

Fig. 14.23 IP needle guidance technique for the anterior sciatic blockade with a needle direction perpendicular to the skin from the lateral side relative to the probe.

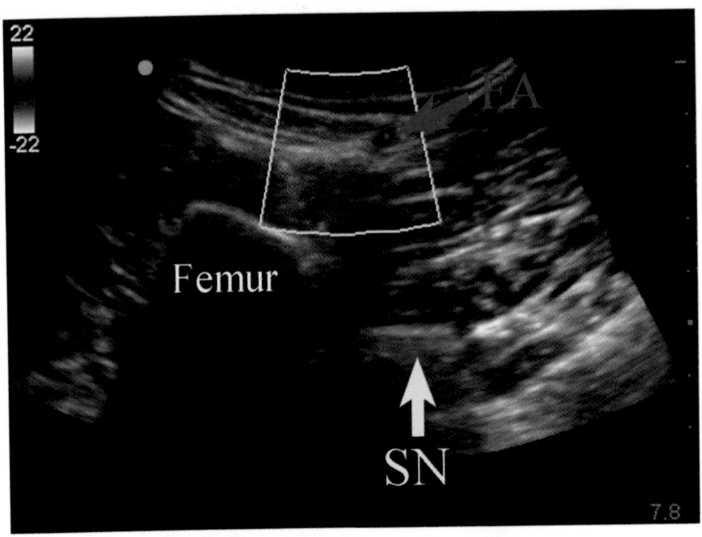

Fig. 14.24 Care should be taken to avoid inadvertent puncture of the femoral artery during the anterior sciatic nerve blockade. FA: femoral artery; SN: sciatic nerve; left side=lateral.

14.7.2.4 Essentials

Block characteristic	Intermediate technique
Patient position	Supine, slightly laterally rotated lower extremity
Ultrasound equipment	Sector probe
Specific ultrasound setting	Low frequency
Important anatomical structures	Minor trochanter, sciatic tuber; rectus femoris, sartorius and greater adductor muscles
Ultrasound appearance of the neuronal structures	Hyperechoic, flat to oval
Expected Vienna score	3–4
Needle equipment	80–120mm, Facette tip
Technique	IP
Estimated local anaesthetic volume	15mL

14.7.3 Subgluteal approach

14.7.3.1 Anatomy (Figure 14.25)

In the subgluteal region, the sciatic nerve is situated between the greater trochanter and the sciatic tuberosity, embedded between the quadriceps femoris

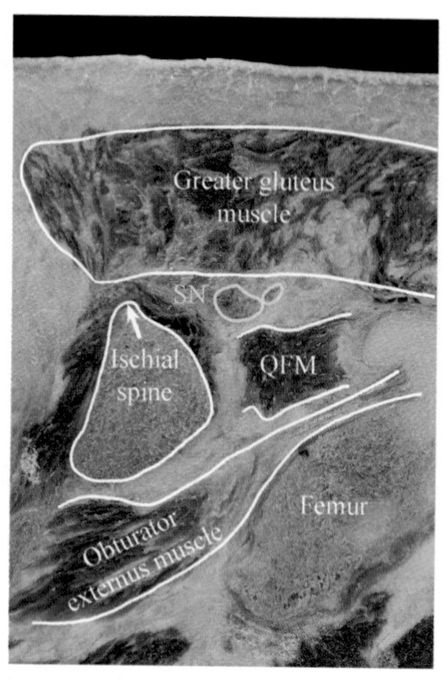

Fig. 14.25 Anatomical cross-sectional view of the sciatic nerve between the greater gluteus muscle and quadratus femoral muscle. SN: sciatic nerve; QFM: quadratus femoral muscle; left side=medial.

and greater gluteus muscles. The cutaneous femoral posterior nerve is found medial to the sciatic nerve in the same layer.

14.7.3.2 Ultrasound guidance technique

The sciatic nerve is in the subgluteal fold in a superficial position and therefore, the blockade under ultrasonographic guidance is attractive. A 38mm linear probe and high frequencies should be used. It appears as flat, oval, hyperechoic nerve structure below the greater gluteus muscle. The cutaneous femoral posterior nerve appears medially to the sciatic nerve as a round and hyperechoic structure (Figure 14.26).

14.7.3.3 Practical block technique

Three patient positions are possible for the practical performance of the subgluteal approach: supine with a 90° flexed hip, lateral position with a 45° flexed hip, or a prone position. An OOP or IP technique can be used (Figure 14.27). Once the tip of the needle is placed laterally to the nerve, the first part of the volume of local anaesthetic is administered. In all cases, it is necessary to redirect the tip of the needle to the medial side of the nerve in order to achieve an adequate spread of the local anaesthetic. In some cases, the sciatic nerve is

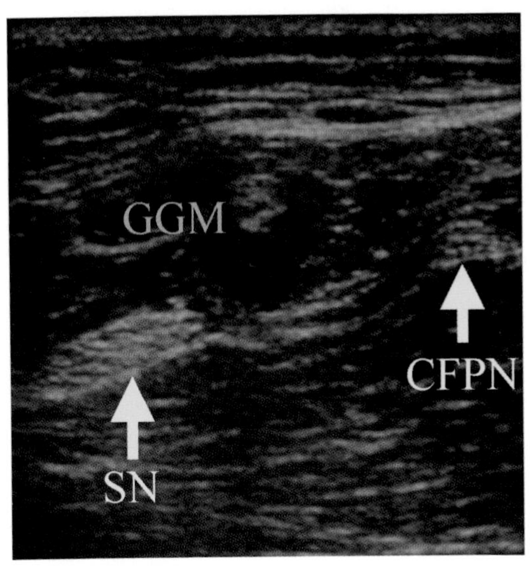

Fig. 14.26 Ultrasonographic appearance of the sciatic and cutaneous femoral posterior nerves at the subgluteal level. SN: sciatic nerve; CFPN: cutaneous femoral posterior nerve; GGM: greater gluteus muscle; left side=lateral.

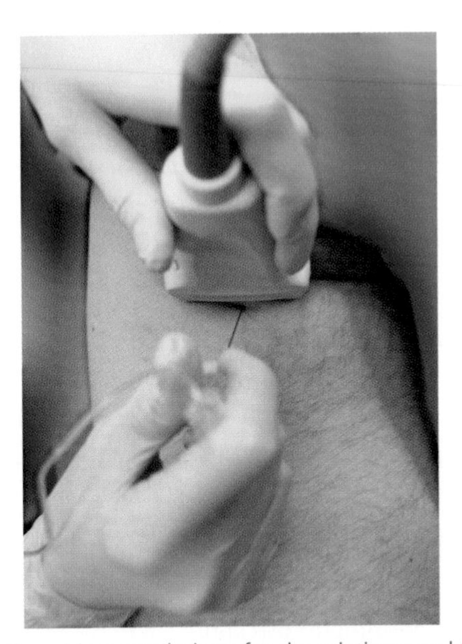

Fig. 14.27 OOP needle guidance technique for the sciatic nerve blockade at the subgluteal level (left side=lateral).

adherent to the quadratus lumborum muscle and therefore, a complete circumferential spread cannot be achieved, which is one explanation for long sensory and motor onset times. By slight medial redirection, additional blockade of the cutaneous femoral posterior nerve can be performed.

14.7.3.4 Essentials

Block characteristic	Intermediate technique
Patient position	Supine, 90° flexed hip and knee Lateral, 45° flexed hip Prone position
Ultrasound equipment	Linear probe, 38mm
Specific ultrasound setting	High to medium frequency
Important anatomical structures	Greater gluteus muscle
Ultrasound appearance of the neuronal structures	Hyperechoic, flat
Expected Vienna score	2
Needle equipment	50mm, Facette tip
Technique	OOP or IP
Estimated local anaesthetic volume	10mL

14.7.4 Mid-femoral approach

14.7.4.1 Anatomy (Figure 14.28)

In the mid-femoral region, the sciatic nerve lies underneath the long head of the biceps muscle. More distally, the nerve is between the long head of the biceps (lateral side of the nerve) and the semitendinosus muscles (medial side of the nerve).

14.7.4.2 Ultrasound guidance technique

The best visibility of the sciatic nerve in the mid-femoral region of the thigh can be achieved between the long head of the biceps and the semitendinosus muscles. A high-frequency, 38mm linear probe should be used and careful probe adjustments provide optimal visibility as a hyperechoic, oval to round structure (Figure 14.29).

14.7.4.3 Practical block technique

Lateral position of the patient with slightly flexed hip and knee is a comfortable and practical patient position for this approach to the sciatic nerve. After visualization of the nerve between the long head of the biceps and semitendinosus

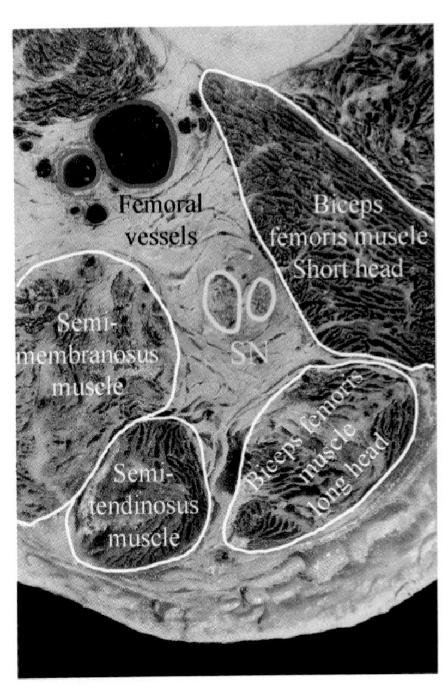

Fig. 14.28 Anatomical cross-sectional view of the thigh at the mid-femoral level with the sciatic nerve between the biceps femoral muscles. SN: sciatic nerve; left side=medial.

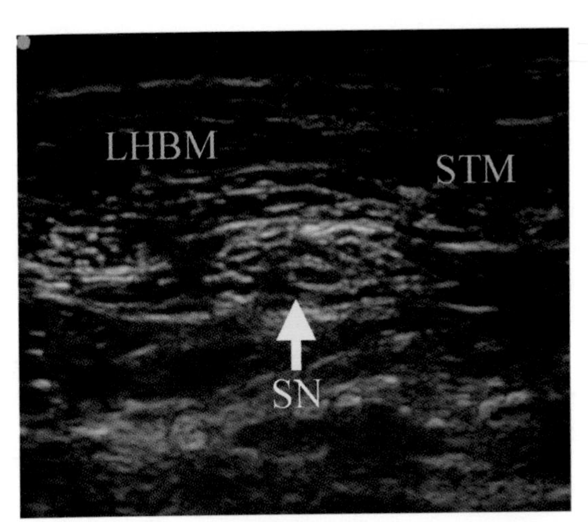

Fig. 14.29 Ultrasonographic appearance of the sciatic nerve at the mid-femoral level. SN: sciatic nerve; LHBM: long head of the biceps muscle; STM: semitendinosus muscle; left side=lateral.

muscles, the needle should be carefully advanced between those two muscles using the OOP or IP technique (Figure 14.30). As described for the more proximal approaches to the sciatic nerve, medial and lateral needle tip position is mandatory for a circumferential spread of local anaesthetic. An alternative technique to block the sciatic nerve from this approach would be with the patient in a prone position and an OOP or IP needle guidance technique.

Figure 14.31 illustrates a large, nutritive vessel supplying the sciatic nerve. We recommend the avoidance of administration of local anaesthetic *plus adrenaline* when such a vessel is recognized.

14.7.4.4 Essentials

Block characteristic	Intermediate technique
Patient position	Lateral or prone
Ultrasound equipment	Linear probe, 38mm
Specific ultrasound setting	High frequency
Important anatomical structures	Long head biceps and semitendinosus muscles
Ultrasound appearance of the neuronal structures	Hyperechoic, oval to round
Expected Vienna score	2
Needle equipment	50–70mm, Facette tip
Technique	OOP or IP
Estimated local anaesthetic volume	6–12mL

14.7.5 **Popliteal approach**

14.7.5.1 Anatomy

In the popliteal area, the sciatic nerve is usually divided into its tibial and common peroneal branches. The main sciatic nerve lies between the biceps femoris (lateral side) and semimembranosus (medial side) muscles, lateral to the popliteal vessels. The common peroneal nerve runs laterally below the lateral head of the gastrocnemius muscle and the tibial nerve runs between the medial and lateral heads of the gastrocnemius muscle to give off the sural nerve (Figure 14.32).

14.7.5.2 Ultrasound guidance technique

Once the sciatic nerve is detected with a high-frequency, linear probe from the popliteal fossa as a hyperechoic, round structure, the nerve should be tracked in a distal direction until the division in its two main branches can be observed

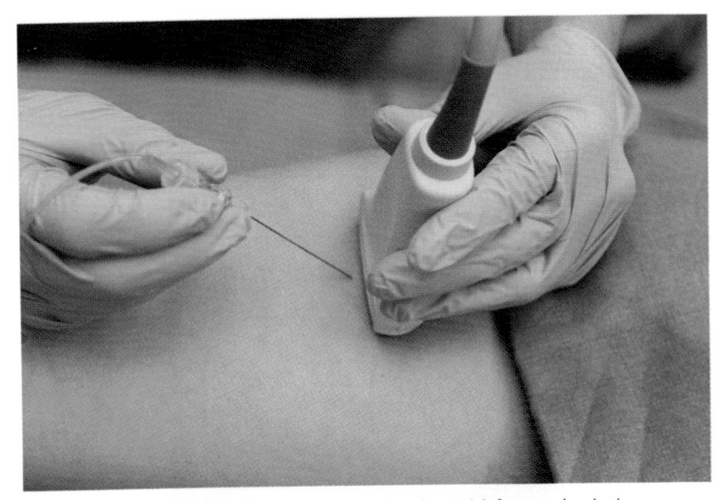

Fig. 14.30 OOP needle guidance technique for the mid-femoral sciatic nerve blockade.

(Figure 14.33). Both the tibial and common peroneus nerves are less echogenic in comparison with the main sciatic nerve.

14.7.5.3 Practical block technique

With the patient in a supine position and the hip and knee flexed, the probe should be placed dorsally to delineate the main sciatic nerve. The block should be performed proximally to the division, except in those cases when a selective blockade of the tibial or common peroneal nerves is required. Once the needle

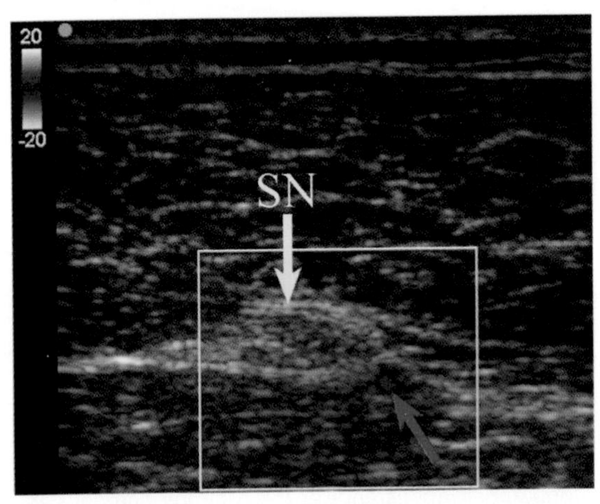

Fig. 14.31 Ultrasound identification of a large nutritive vessel (red arrow) supplying the sciatic nerve (SN).

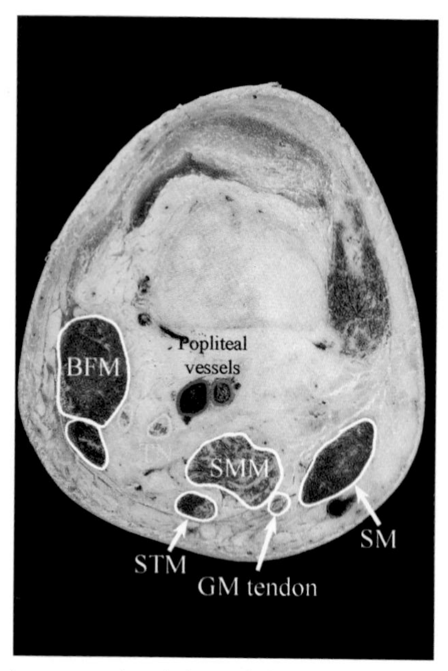

Fig. 14.32 Anatomical cross-sectional view of the thigh at the popliteal level. CPN: common peroneus nerve; TN: tibial nerve; BFM: biceps femoris muscle; GM: gracilis muscle; STM: semitendinosus muscle; SMM: semimembranosus muscle; SM: sartorius muscle; left side=lateral.

is introduced below the biceps femoris muscle, the tip should be placed using the IP technique above and below the nerve to achieve a circumferential spread of local anaesthetic (Figures 14.34 and 14.35). The techniques to block the tibial and common peroneal nerves are identical. An alternative technique to

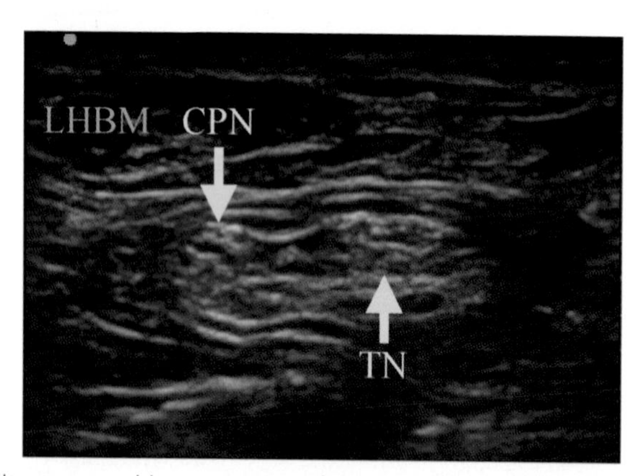

Fig. 14.33 Ultrasonographic appearance of the common peroneus and tibial nerves slightly distal to the sciatic nerve division. CPN: common peroneus nerve; TN: tibial nerve; LHBM: long head of the biceps femoral muscle; left side=lateral.

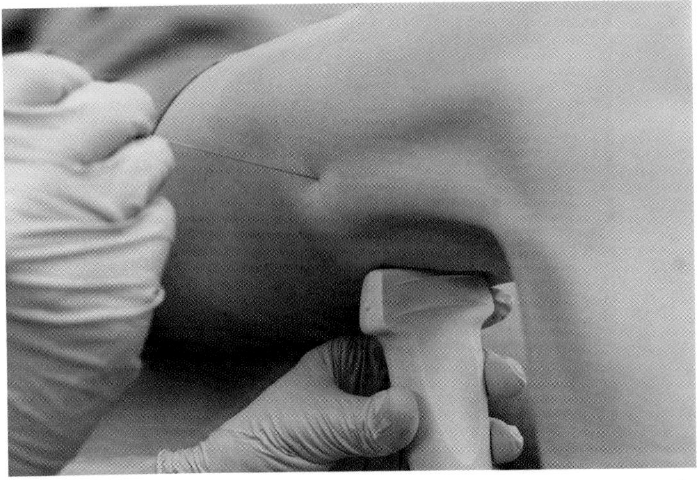

Fig. 14.34 IP needle guidance technique for blockade of the sciatic nerve at the popliteal level.

block the sciatic nerve from this approach would be in prone position with an OOP or IP technique.

14.7.5.4 Essentials

Block characteristic	Intermediate technique
Patient position	Supine, hip and knee flexed, pillow under the ankle
Ultrasound equipment	Linear probe, 38mm
Specific ultrasound setting	High frequency
Important anatomical structures	Biceps femoris and semimembranosus muscles, popliteal vessels
Ultrasound appearance of the neuronal structures	Main sciatic nerve: hyperechoic, round Tibial and common peroneal nerves: less hyperechoic in comparison to sciatic nerve, round
Expected Vienna score	Main sciatic nerve: 2 Tibial and common peroneal nerves: 3
Needle equipment	70–100mm, Facette tip
Technique	IP
Estimated local anaesthetic volume	8–12mL

14.8 **Ankle blocks**

Ankle blocks are very popular for foot surgery, but the descriptions of those blocks are purely based on superficial anatomical landmarks. To compensate for those weak descriptions, relatively large volumes of local anaesthetics

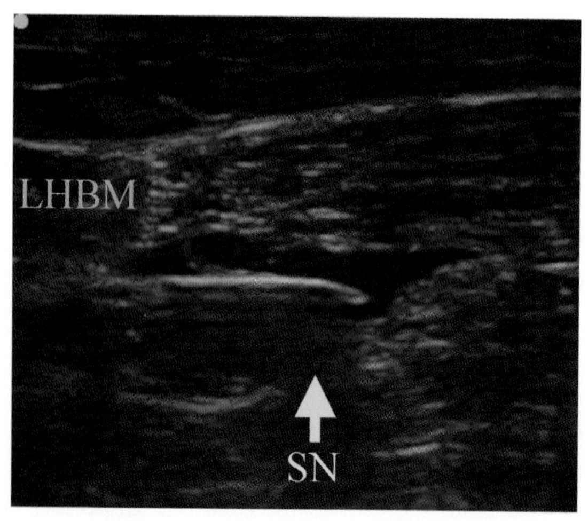

Fig. 14.35 IP needle guidance technique for the sciatic nerve blockade at the popliteal level, slightly proximal to the division (large parts of the sciatic nerve are hidden by the body of the needle). SN: sciatic nerve; LHBM: long head of the biceps femoral muscle; left side=lateral.

are recommended for these techniques with subsequent pain during injection due to the fact that tense tendons and muscles are in a close proximity to the nerves. None of these blocks are described in sufficient scientific manner in the literature.

Usually, blockade of the tibial and deep and superficial branches of the peroneus nerves are necessary for most types of foot surgery.

14.8.1 Tibial nerve

14.8.1.1 Anatomy

The tibial nerve passes posteriorly to the medial malleolus closely adjacent to the posterior tibial artery and vein. The tendons of the tibialis posterior and flexor digitorum longus muscles are situated anteriorly to the nerve. Posterior to the tibial nerve lies the tendon of the flexor hallucis longus muscle (Figure 14.36).

14.8.1.2 Anatomical variations

Variations in the arrangement of the tibial nerve around the vessels are possible.

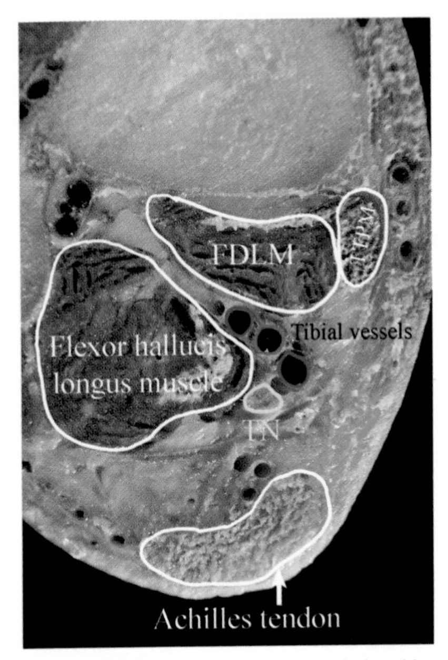

Fig. 14.36 Anatomical cross-sectional view of the medial ankle with the tibial nerve. TN: tibial nerve; FDLM: flexor digitorum longus muscle; TTPM: tendon of the tibialis posterior muscle; left side=medial.

14.8.1.3 Ultrasound guidance technique

The optimal position of the 25mm high-frequency, linear probe is slightly proximal to the medial malleolus. The major landmark is the posterior tibial artery; the nerve can be visualized as hyperechoic, round structure close to the artery (Figure 14.37).

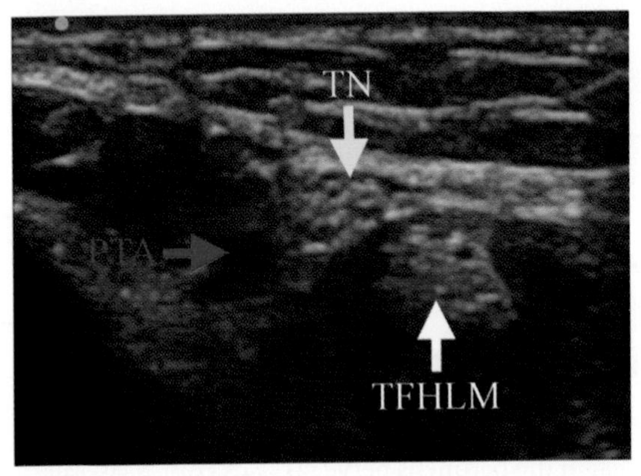

Fig. 14.37 Ultrasonographic appearance of the tibial nerve slightly cranial to the medial malleolus. TN: tibial nerve; PTA: posterior tibial artery; TFHLM: tendon of the flexor hallucis longus muscle; left side=anterior.

14.8.1.4 Practical block technique

After optimal visualization of the tibial nerve slightly proximal to the medial malleolus, the block should be performed using the OOP technique (Figure 14.38) and a small volume of local anaesthetic. Prior to the block, careful aspiration is mandatory since several veins are located around the nerve.

14.8.1.5 Essentials

Block characteristic	Basic technique
Patient position	Supine, externally rotated lower leg
Ultrasound equipment	Linear probe, 25mm
Specific ultrasound setting	High frequency
Important anatomical structures	Posterior tibial artery
Ultrasound appearance of the neuronal structures	Hyperechoic, round
Expected Vienna score	2
Needle equipment	30–50mm, Facette tip
Technique	OOP
Estimated local anaesthetic volume	1–2mL

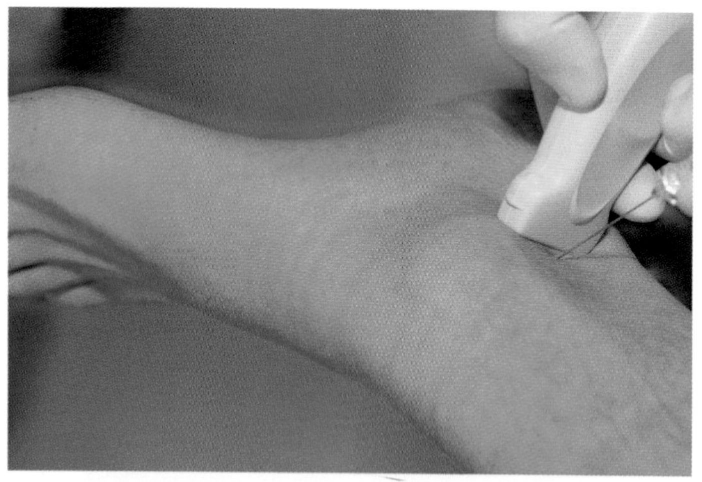

Fig. 14.38 OOP needle guidance technique to block the tibial nerve slightly cranial to the medial malleolus.

14.8.2 Deep branch of the peroneus nerve

14.8.2.1 Anatomy

The deep branch of the peroneus nerve takes its course laterally to the anterior tibial artery in a distal direction.

14.8.2.2 Anatomical variations

The absence of this branch and replacement of innervation by the saphenous and sural nerves have been described.

14.8.2.3 Ultrasound guidance technique

The high-frequency, linear probe should be placed on the medial lateral side of the distal lower leg. The nerve can be detected using a high-frequency, linear probe between the extensor hallucis longus and extensor digitorum longus muscles as hyperechoic, round structure (Figure 14.39).

14.8.2.4 Practical block technique

The block should be performed using the OOP technique with the needle direction between the extensor hallucis longus and extensor digitorum longus muscles (Figure 14.40). Care should be taken to avoid puncture of the anterior tibial artery.

14.8.2.5 Essentials

Block characteristic	Basic technique
Patient position	Supine, neutral leg position
Ultrasound equipment	Linear probe, 25–38mm
Specific ultrasound setting	High frequency
Important anatomical structures	Anterior tibial artery
Ultrasound appearance of the neuronal structures	Hyperechoic, round
Expected Vienna score	2
Needle equipment	50mm, Facette tip
Technique	OOP
Estimated local anaesthetic volume	1–2mL

14.8.3 Superficial branch of the peroneus nerve

14.8.3.1 Anatomy

The superficial branch of the peroneal nerve runs at the mid-level of the lower leg between the short and long fibular muscles on the lateral side. Above the lateral malleolus, the nerve is in a very superficial position above the deep fascia which forms the superior extensor retinaculum.

14.8.3.2 Anatomical variations

The absence of this nerve and replacement of innervation by the saphenous and sural nerves have been described.

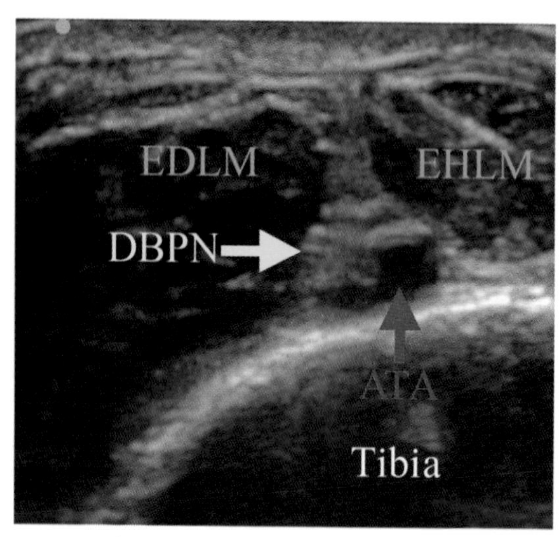

Fig. 14.39 Ultrasonographic appearance of the deep branch of the peroneus nerve close to the anterior tibial artery between the extensor tibialis. DBPN: deep branch of the peroneus nerve; ATA: anterior tibial artery; EDLM: extensor digitorum longus muscle; EHLM: extensor hallucis longus muscle; left side=lateral.

14.8.3.3 Ultrasound guidance technique

On placing the high-frequency, linear probe cranial and anterior to the lateral malleolus, the nerve appears as a small, hyperechoic, round structure (Figure 14.41). The identification may be difficult due to the lack of clear landmarks.

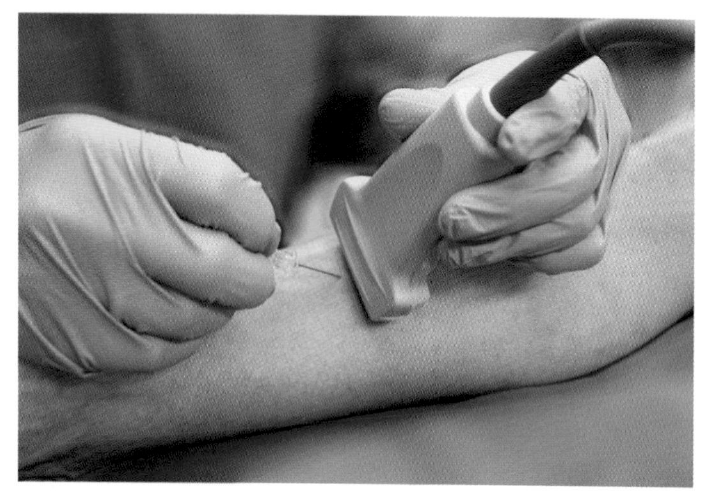

Fig. 14.40 OOP needle guidance technique for blockade of the deep branch of the peroneus nerve.

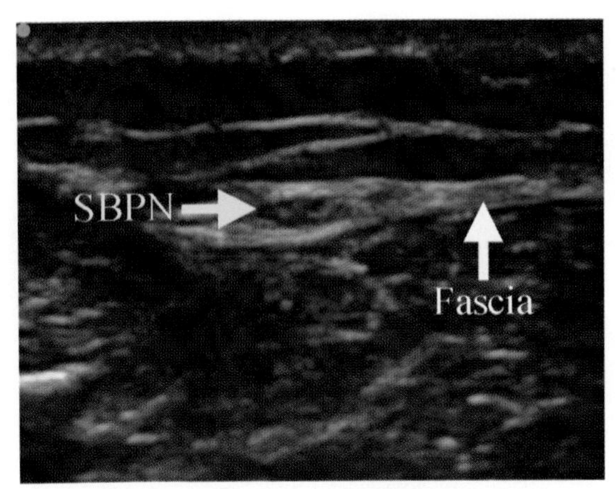

Fig. 14.41 Ultrasonographic appearance of the superficial branch of the peroneus nerve where it pierces the fascia. SBPN: superficial branch of the peroneus nerve; left side=lateral.

14.8.3.4 Practical block technique

Once the nerve is identified, an OOP technique should be performed to block the nerve (Figure 14.42). In cases of difficulties in the safe identification of the nerve, a more proximal approach should be used.

14.8.3.5 Essentials

Block characteristic	Basic technique
Patient position	Supine, neutral leg position
Ultrasound equipment	Linear probe, 25mm
Specific ultrasound setting	High frequency
Important anatomical structures	–
Ultrasound appearance of the neuronal structures	Hyperechoic, round
Expected Vienna score	2–3
Technique	OOP
Needle equipment	50mm, Facette tip
Estimated local anaesthetic volume	1–2mL

14.9 **Implications of lower limb blocks in children**

Peripheral lower limb blocks are absolutely underused in children. In most children under 25kg body weight, caudal blocks can be used for surgery of the lower limbs. For children over 25kg body weight, peripheral block techniques of the lumbosacral plexus can be extremely useful. Similar to upper limb blocks, all

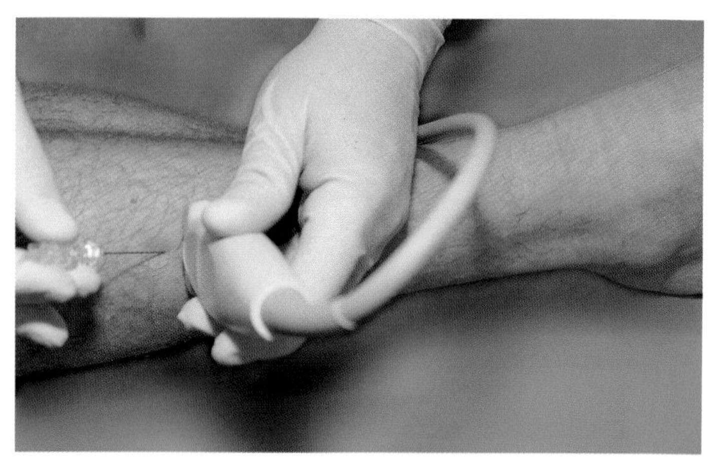

Fig. 14.42 OOP needle guidance for blockade of the superficial branch of the peroneus nerve.

blocks of the lower limbs in adults as described above are applicable in children. Due to the fact that in most cases, nerve structures are more superficial than in the adult population, the block techniques are easier to perform. A 24G Facette tip needle should be used in children under 10kg whereas a 22G Facette tip needle should be used in children over 10kg. The volumes of local anaesthetics should be also adjusted to the reduced cross-sectional areas of nerves in children.

Peripheral nerve blocks may be also useful in extreme weight groups in cases of lack of alternatives. Figures 14.43 and 14.44 illustrate a sciatic nerve

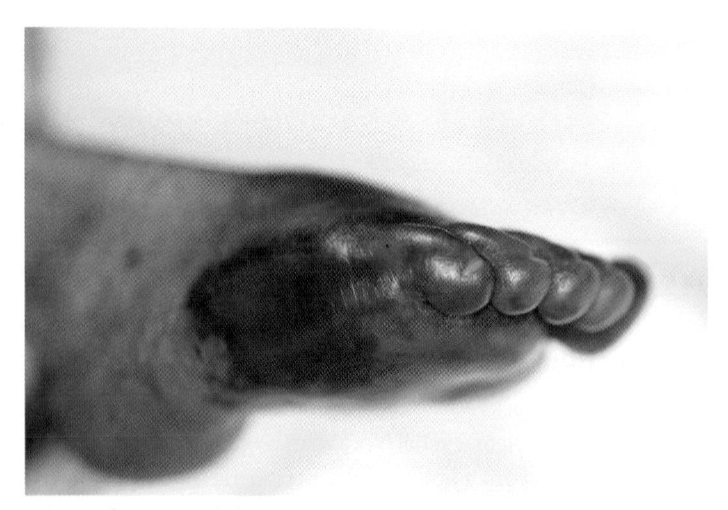

Fig. 14.43 Forefoot necrosis in a 1,021g neonate after a feto-fetal transfusion syndrome.

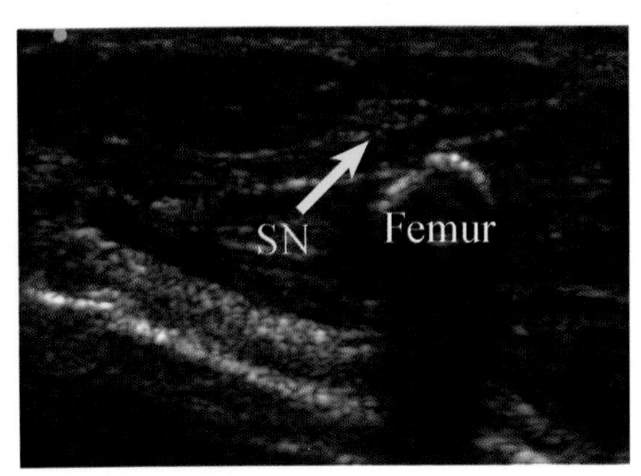

Fig. 14.44 Ultrasound illustration of the sciatic nerve (SN) in a 1,021g neonate prior to blockade for therapeutic sympatholysis.

blockade as therapeutic sympatholysis for a case of forefoot necrosis in a 1,021g anticoagulated neonate.

Suggested further reading

Chan, V., Nova, H., Abbas, S., McCartney, C., Perlas, A., Xu, D., 2006. Ultrasound examination and localization of the sciatic nerve: a volunteer study. *Anesthesiology*, 104(2), pp.309–14.

Hurdle, M., Weingarten, T., Crisostomo, R., Psimos, C., Smith, J., 2007. Ultrasound-guided blockade of the lateral femoral cutaneous nerve: technical description and review of 10 cases. *Archives of Physical Medicine and Rehabilitation*, 88(10), pp.1362–4.

Karmakar, M.K., Kwok, W.H., Ho, A.M., Tsang, K., Chui, P.T., Gin, T., 2007. Ultrasound-guided sciatic nerve block: description of a new approach at the subgluteal space. *British Journal of Anaesthesia*, 98(3), pp.390–5.

Kirchmair, L., Entner, T., Kapral, S., Mitterschiffthaler, G., 2002. Ultrasound guidance for the psoas compartment block: an imaging study. *Anesthesia & Analgesia*, 94(3), pp.706–10.

Latzke, D., Marhofer, P., Zeitlinger, M., Machata, A., Neumann, F., Lackner, E., Kettner, S.C., 2010. Minimal local anaesthetic volumes for sciatic nerve block: evaluation of ED99 in volunteers. *British Journal of Anaesthesia*, 104(2), pp.239–44.

Lundblad, M., Kapral, S., Marhofer, P., Lönnqvist, P.A., 2006. Ultrasound-guided infrapatellar nerve block in human volunteers: description of a novel technique. *British Journal of Anaesthesia*, 97(5), pp.710–4.

Marhofer, P., Schrögendorfer, K., Koinig, H., Kapral, S., Weinstabl, C., Mayer, N., 1997. Ultrasonographic guidance improves sensory block and onset time of three-in-one blocks. *Anesthesia & Analgesia*, 85(4), pp.854–7.

Marhofer, P., Schrögendorfer, K., Wallner, T., Koinig, H., Mayer, N., Kapral, S., 1998. Ultrasonographic guidance reduces the amount of local anaesthetic for 3-in-1 blocks. *Regional Anesthesia and Pain Medicine*, 23(6), pp.584–8.

Oberndorfer, U., Marhofer, P., Bösenberg, A., Willschke, H., Felfernig, M., Weintraud, M., Kapral, S., Kettner, S.C., 2007. Ultrasonographic guidance for sciatic and femoral nerve blocks in children. *British Journal of Anaesthesia*, 98(6), pp.797–801.

Soong, J., Schaffhalter–Zoppoth, I., Gray, A., 2007. Sonographic imaging of the obturator nerve for regional block. *Regional Anesthesia and Pain Medicine*, 32(2), pp.146–51.

Chapter 15

Truncal blocks

15.1 General anatomical considerations

Truncal blocks are well established, regional, anaesthetic techniques in the thoracic and abdominal regions, providing pain relief by blocking the sensory end branches of the ventral rami T7–12 and L1–3. Historically, blind techniques relying on tactile sensation ('scratching sensations' or 'palpable gives') to identify the correct needle position have been the standard method for these nerve blocks. These simple, but often forgotten, blocks can be divided into four techniques:

- *Intercostal nerve blocks* provide analgesia for thoracic and upper abdominal surgery. Blockade of two dermatomes above and two below the level of surgery is required for an adequate analgesia.
- *Ilioinguinal/iliohypogastric* nerve blocks are common analgesic techniques for providing adequate pain relief during inguinal surgery.
- *Rectus sheath blocks* provide effective pain relief for umbilical or other midline surgical approaches. This regional anaesthetic technique was first described by Schleich in 1899 to provide relaxation of the anterior abdominal wall by blocking the terminal branches of intercostal nerves 9–11 within the rectus sheath.
- *Transversus abdominis plane blocks* provide simultaneous blockade of the T7–12 intercostal nerves, the ilioinguinal and iliohypogastric nerves, and the lateral cutaneous branches of the dorsal rami of L1–3.

15.2 Intercostal blocks

15.2.1 Anatomy

The intercostal nerves supply the skin and the muscles of the chest and abdominal wall. They can be visualized at the dorsum of the thorax and between the pleura and posterior intercostal membrane. After a short distance, they pierce the posterior intercostal membrane and run between the two planes of the intercostal muscles. After approximately two-thirds of their course, the intercostal nerves pass within the fibres of the intercostales interni muscles. As they approach the costal cartilages, the nerves reach the inner surface of the intercostales interni muscles and subsequently run below the pleura. Finally, the intercostal nerves pass inferior to their respective rib, together with the intercostal vessels (Figure 15.1).

15.2.2 Anatomical variations

Thoracic spinal roots as well as the ventral rami may be absent.

15.2.3 Ultrasound guidance technique

Due to the sonic shadow of the rib, it is usually not possible to visualize the intercostal nerves. It is therefore essential to define the external and internal intercostal muscles and the pleura (Figure 15.2). The puncture should be performed at the level of the posterior axillary line. Administration of 1.5mL of local anaesthetic is usually sufficient when administered within the internal intercostal muscle to fill up the entire intercostal space. With this amount of local anaesthetic, it is also possible to block the collateral branch on the upper border of the caudal rib.

15.2.4 Practical block technique

After the exact identification of the ribs, the external and internal intercostal muscles, and the pleura in the posterior axillary line, the needle is inserted by the OOP technique with the transducer positioned transversely to the ribs

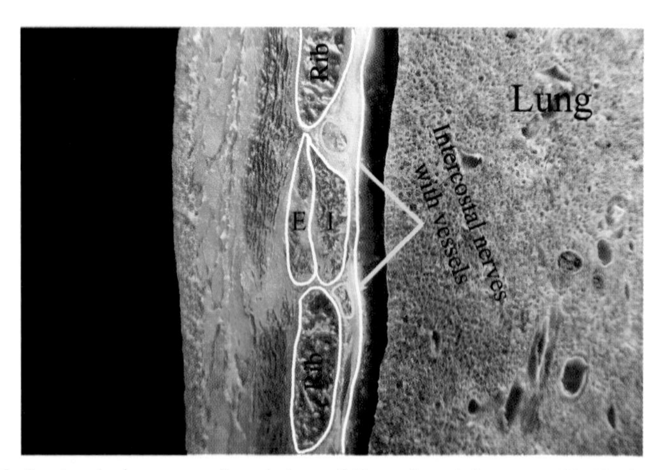

Fig. 15.1 Anatomical cross-sectional view of the subcostal space with the intercostal nerves and vessels. E: external intercostal muscle; I: internal intercostal muscle.

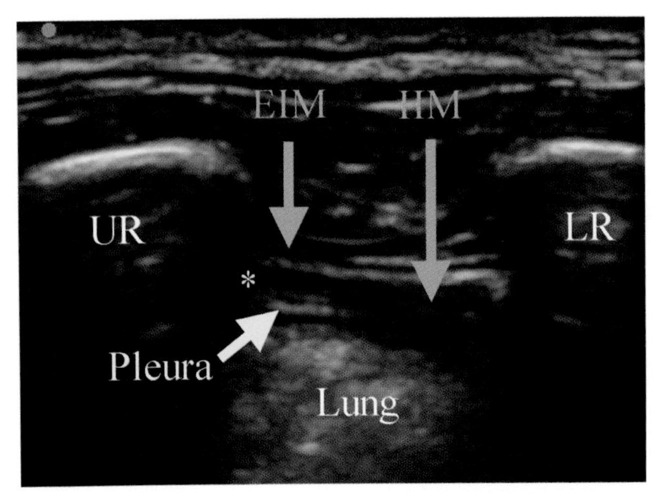

Fig. 15.2 Ultrasonographic identification of the external and internal intercostal muscles and pleura. EIM: external intercostal muscle; IIM: internal intercostal muscle; UR: upper rib; LR: lower rib; * indicates the injection point of local anaesthetic; left side=cranial.

(Figure 15.3). The needle should be inserted very carefully into the external intercostal muscle. The correct position of the tip of the needle within the external intercostal muscle can be verified by injecting very small amounts (0.2mL) of local anaesthetic. Once verified, the needle should be advanced carefully within the internal intercostal muscle and upon correct positioning, a total of 1.5mL of local anaesthetic is injected.

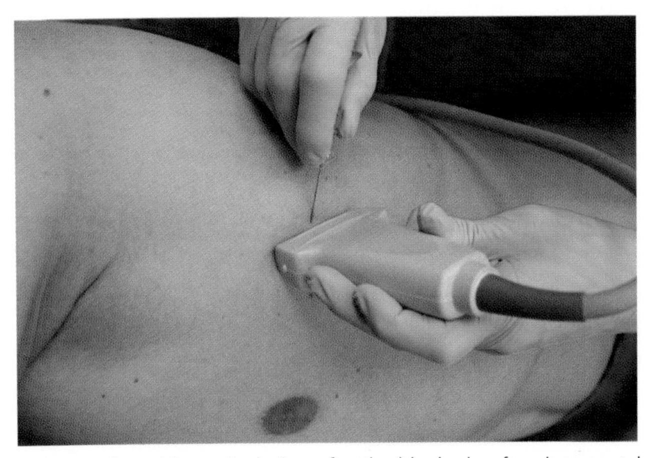

Fig. 15.3 OOP needle guidance technique for the blockade of an intercostal nerve.

15.2.5 Essentials

Block characteristic	Basic technique
Patient position	Supine, thorax slightly laterally rotated
Ultrasound equipment	Linear probe, 38mm
Specific ultrasound setting	High frequency
Important anatomical structures	External and internal intercostal muscle, pleura
Ultrasound appearance of the neuronal structures	–
Expected Vienna score	–
Needle equipment	50mm, Facette tip
Needle guidance technique	OOP
Estimated local anaesthetic volume	1.5mL

15.3 Ilioinguinal-iliohypogastric nerve blocks

15.3.1 Anatomy

The iliohypogastric nerve is formed by the ventral ramus L1 and a branch of T12. It emerges from the lateral border of the psoas major muscle, passes across the ventral surface of the quadratus lumborum, and descends to the iliac crest. As it approaches the anterior superior iliac spine, the nerve pierces the transverse abdominal muscle to take its course beneath the internal oblique and transverse abdominal muscles (Figure 15.4). The ilioinguinal nerve, which is formed by the ventral rami L1–2, follows a similar course.

15.3.2 Anatomical variations

Both nerves occasionally arise as a common trunk, only to become separated between the transverse and internal oblique muscles. The iliohypogastric nerve sometimes arises from the subcostal nerve; it may also receive a branch from the 11th thoracic nerve. In some cases, the ilioinguinal nerve may terminate near the iliac crest to join the iliohypogastric nerve, whereupon branches of the iliohypogastric nerve replace the absent fibres. A lateral cutaneous or iliac branch may arise to supply the skin in the region of the anterior superior iliac spine. It may also replace the genital branch of the genitofemoral nerve or the lateral femoral cutaneous nerve. In rare cases, the ilioinguinal nerve is absent altogether.

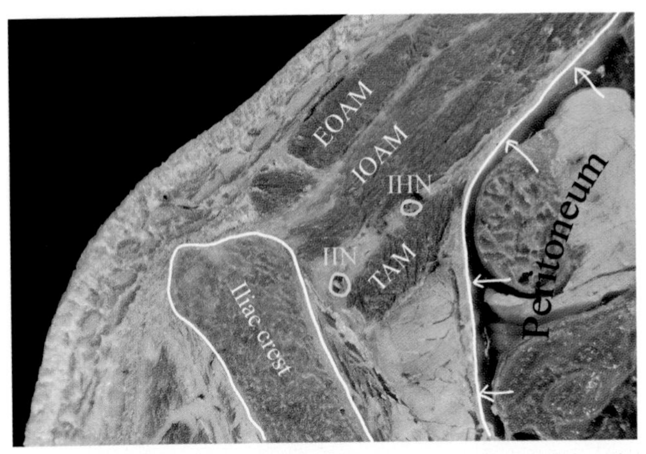

Fig. 15.4 Anatomical cross-sectional view of the inguinal area medial to the superior iliac spine. IHN: iliohypogastric nerve; IIN: ilioinguinal nerve; EOAM: external oblique abdominal muscle; IOAM: internal oblique abdominal muscle; TAM: transverse abdominal muscle; left=lateral.

15.3.3 Ultrasound guidance technique

In adults, the ilioinguinal and iliohypogastric nerves are best visible 1–2cm cranial and lateral to the anterior superior iliac spine. Here, the nerves can usually be found situated between the internal oblique abdominal muscle and the transverse abdominal muscle. Figure 15.5 shows a typical ultrasound picture of this region. The position of the ultrasound probe is transverse in relation to the nerves.

15.3.4 Practical block technique

After the identification of the ilioinguinal and iliohypogastric nerves, the block is performed using the OOP technique. In general, it is possible to place the tip of the needle between the ilioinguinal and iliohypogastric nerves and inject 0.1mL/kg of local anaesthetic to achieve an adequate distribution. In patients with chronic pain, it is possible to distinguish whether a pain syndrome is caused by either the iliohypogastric or ilioinguinal nerve by blocking each nerve with 1mL of local anaesthetic. For this purpose, the diffusion of local anaesthetic along a fascial plane should be avoided. Figures 15.6 and 15.7 illustrate the OOP needle guidance technique and a typical ultrasound picture of the puncture site after injection. The needle is placed in between both nerves. Care should be taken to avoid puncturing the large vessels of the abdominal wall (e.g. profound circumflexa ilium artery) (Figure 15.8).

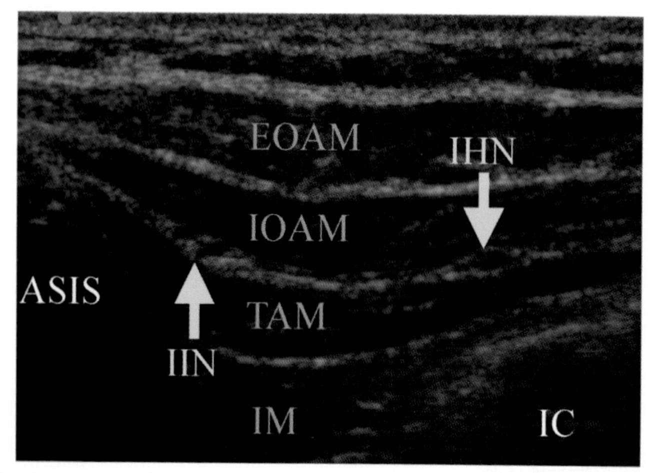

Fig. 15.5 Ultrasonographic illustration of the lateral abdominal wall at the level of the anterior superior iliac spine. IIN: ilioinguinal nerve; IHN: iliohypogastric nerve; ASIS: anterior superior iliac spine; EOAM: external oblique abdominal muscle; IOAM: internal oblique abdominal muscle; TAM: transverse abdominal muscle; IM: iliac muscle; IC: intraperitoneal cavum; left side=lateral.

15.3.5 Essentials

Block characteristic	Basic technique
Patient position	Supine
Ultrasound equipment	Linear probe, 38mm
Specific ultrasound setting	High frequency
Important anatomical structures	External oblique, internal oblique, and transverse abdominal muscles
Ultrasound appearance of the neuronal structures	Round and oval hyperechoic nerves
Expected Vienna score	1–2
Needle equipment	50mm, Facette tip
Needle guidance technique	OOP
Estimated local anaesthetic volume	0.1mL/kg

15.4 Rectus sheath block

15.4.1 Anatomy

The central abdominal wall consists of the rectus abdominal muscle, which is embedded in the anterior and posterior rectus sheath. These fascial sheaths are formed by the aponeurosis of the transverse, internal oblique, and external

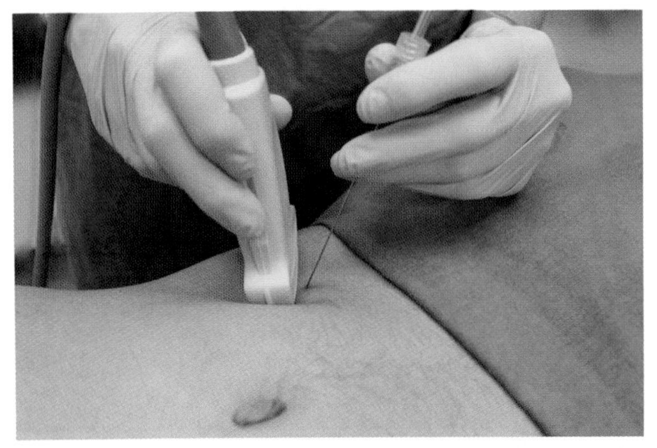

Fig. 15.6 OOP needle guidance technique for blockade of the ilioinguinal/iliohypogastric nerves.

oblique abdominal muscles. There are three tendinous intersections within the rectus abdominis muscle, one at the level of the xiphoid, one at the umbilicus, and one in between. The intercostal nerves 9–11 pass behind the costal cartilage and between the internal oblique and transversus abdominis muscle. Usually, the nerves run between the posterior rectus sheath and the posterior wall of the rectus abdominis muscle. Ultimately, they perforate the sheath with their anterior cutaneous branches supplying the skin in the midline (Figure 15.9).

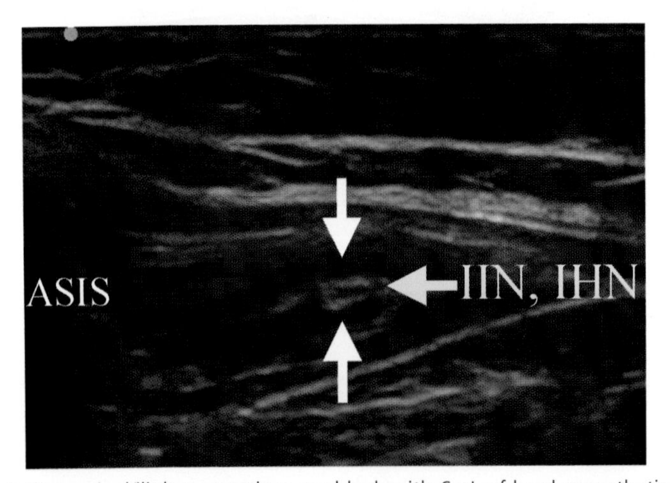

Fig. 15.7 Ilioinguinal/iliohypogastric nerve block with 6mL of local anaesthetic (white arrows). IIN & IHN: ilioinguinal and iliohypogastric nerves; left side=lateral.

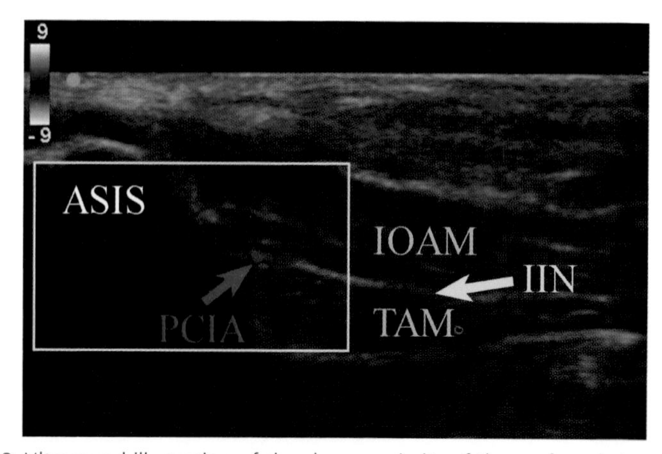

Fig. 15.8 Ultrasound illustration of the close proximity of the profound circumflexa ilium artery to the ilioinguinal nerve medial to the anterior superior iliac spine and between the internal oblique and transverse abdominal muscles. PCIA: profound circumflexa ilium artery; IIN: ilioinguinal nerve; ASIS: anterior superior iliac spine; IOAM: internal oblique abdominal muscle; TAM: transverse abdominal muscle; left=lateral.

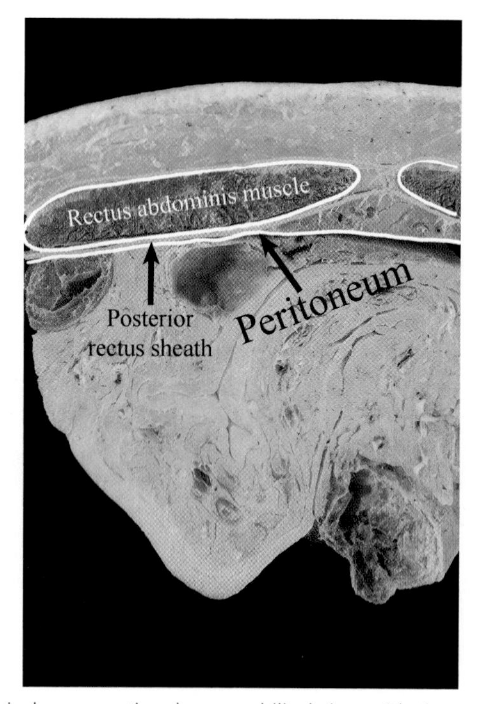

Fig. 15.9 Anatomical cross-sectional paraumbilical view with the posterior rectus sheath (left=lateral).

15.4.2 Anatomical variations

It has been reported that parts or even the whole of the rectus abdominis muscle may be absent or doubled. Numerous variations concerning the origins and insertions of the abdominal muscles have been described, but seem to have no impact on the described technique of rectus sheath block.

15.4.3 Ultrasound guidance technique

The main difference to most other peripheral regional anaesthetic techniques is that the local anaesthetic is injected next to a fascial plane without direct visualization of the nerve structures. Diffusion along this plane will lead the local anaesthetic to the terminal branches of the intercostal nerves. Using ultrasonography, it is possible to place the local anaesthetic in between the posterior rectus sheath and the rectus abdominis muscle. We recommend placing the ultrasound probe in a transverse position in relation to the rectus abdominal muscle.

15.4.4 Practical block technique

After the exact identification of the rectus abdominis muscle and the posterior rectus sheath, the block is performed bilaterally at the level of the umbilicus using an OOP technique (Figures 15.10 and 15.11). Once the tip of the needle is correctly positioned between the rectus abdominis muscle and the posterior rectus sheath, a predetermined volume of 0.1mL/kg of local anaesthetic is injected (Figure 15.12).

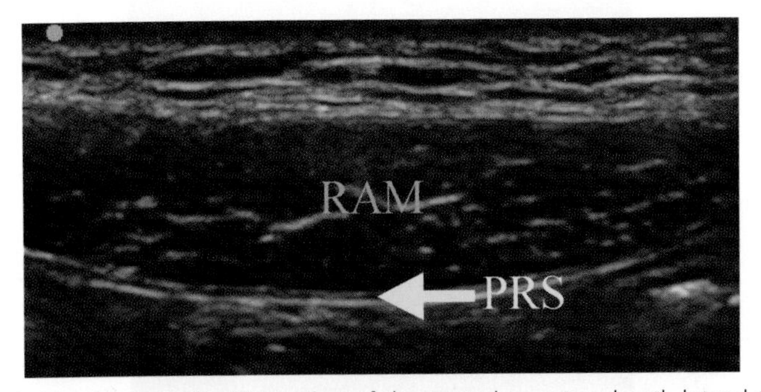

Fig. 15.10 Ultrasonographic illustration of the posterior rectus sheath lateral to the umbilicus.PRS: posterior rectus sheath; RAM: rectus abdominis muscle; left side=lateral.

15.4.5 Essentials

Block characteristic	Basic technique
Patient position	Supine
Ultrasound equipment	Linear probe
Specific ultrasound setting	High frequency
Important anatomical structures	Rectus abdominis muscle, anterior and posterior rectus sheath
Ultrasound appearance of the neuronal structures	–
Expected Vienna score	–
Needle equipment	50mm, Facette tip
Needle guidance technique	OOP
Estimated local anaesthetic volume	0.1mL/kg/side

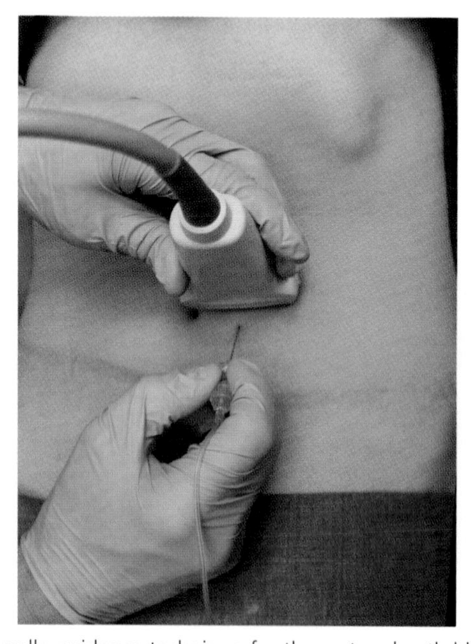

Fig. 15.11 OOP needle guidance technique for the rectus sheath block.

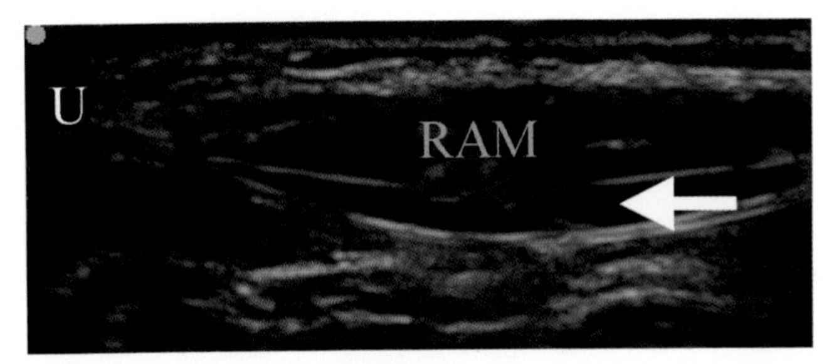

Fig. 15.12 Rectus sheath block with 0.1mL/kg of local anaesthetic (white arrow). RAM: rectus abdominis muscle; U: umbilicus; left side=medial.

15.5 Transversus abdominis plane (TAP) block

15.5.1 Anatomy

The lateral abdominal wall contains the following nerves: T7–12 intercostal nerves, the ilioinguinal and iliohypogastric nerves, the lateral cutaneous branches of the dorsal rami of L1–3.

The intercostal nerves, subcostal nerves, and first lumbar nerves that contribute to the innervation of the anterior abdominal wall run in a neurovascular plane known as the transversus abdominis plane which is located between the internal oblique and transversus abdominis muscles.

15.5.2 Anatomical variations

The anatomical relationship of the nerves is highly individual. Extensive branching and communication of the nerves within the transversus abdominis plane is possible.

15.5.3 Ultrasound guidance technique

The lateral abdominal wall can be scanned with a high/medium frequency, linear ultrasound probe. The identification of the external oblique, internal oblique, and transverse abdominal muscles should be possible without problems.

15.5.4 Practical block technique

With the patient in a supine position, the ultrasound scan should be performed between the iliac crest and the 12th rib. Using an IP needle guidance technique as illustrated in Figure 15.13, the tip of the needle needs to be placed between the internal oblique and transverse abdominal muscles, and a predetermined volume of 20mL of local anaesthetic is recommended to be administered (Figure 15.14). The needle visibility is impaired due to the steep

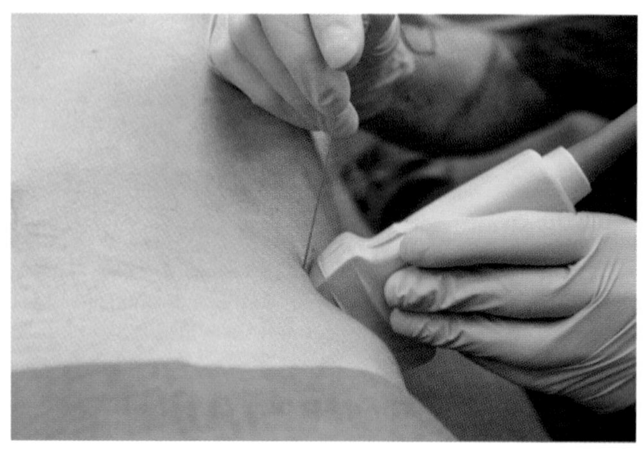

Fig. 15.13 IP needle guidance technique for TAP blockade.

angle of insertion. As described above, current developments in needle technology also provide improved visibility of needles for steep angles during the IP needle guidance technique.

If a bilateral block is required, the same procedure needs to be performed on the contralateral side.

15.5.5 Essentials

Block characteristic	Basic technique
Patient position	Supine
Ultrasound equipment	Linear probe
Specific ultrasound setting	High frequency
Important anatomical structures	External oblique, internal oblique, and transversal abdominal muscles
Ultrasound appearance of the neuronal structures	–
Expected Vienna score	–
Needle equipment	70–90mm, Facette tip
Needle guidance technique	IP
Estimated local anaesthetic volume	20mL/side

15.6 Implications of truncal blocks in children

Ultrasound-guided truncal blocks in children are well investigated. Our study group described in several publications the performance of ilioinguinal-iliohypogastric and rectus sheath blocks. The initial description of *ilioinguinal-iliohypogastric blocks* was based on a randomized and comparative study in

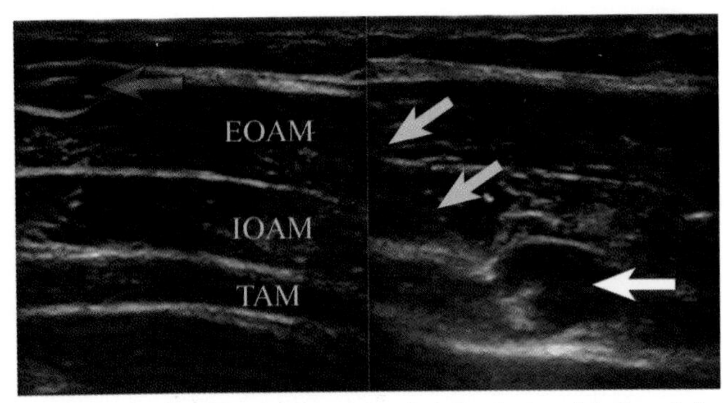

Fig. 15.14 Ultrasound illustration of the lateral abdominal wall before (left side) and after administration of local anaesthetic (right side) during an IP needle guidance technique. The transparent arrow in the left image indicates the skin wheal; the grey arrows in the right image indicate the body of the needle. EOAM: external oblique abdominal muscle; IOAM: internal oblique abdominal muscle; TAM: transverse abdominal muscle; left side in both parts of the figure=cranial.

100 children with a success rate of 96% in the ultrasound group compared with a 74% success rate in the 'fascial click' group. The ultrasound-guided technique is easy to perform with either an IP or OOP technique. The identification of the ilioinguinal and iliohypogastric nerves is usually simple at the level of the anterior superior iliac spine between the internal oblique and transversus abdominis muscles (Figure 15.15). It is important to note that the external oblique abdominal muscle is frequently only available as an aponeurosis in children. In a subsequent study, a local anaesthetic volume of

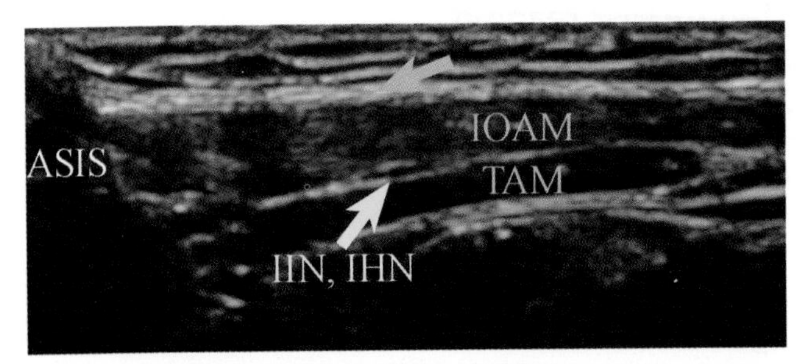

Fig. 15.15 Ultrasound illustration of the ilioinguinal/iliohypogastric nerves medial to the anterior superior iliac spine and between the internal oblique and transverse abdominal muscles in a 5kg baby. The arrow indicates the aponeurosis of the external oblique abdominal muscle. IIN: ilioinguinal nerve; IHN: iliohypogastric nerve; ASIS: anterior superior iliac spine; IOAM: internal oblique abdominal muscle; TAM: transverse abdominal muscle; left side=lateral.

0.075mL/kg was found to be sufficient for this regional anaesthetic technique by using a new volume reduction protocol, which seems to be important because the ultrasound-guided technique is associated with higher plasma levels of local anaesthetics compared with the conventional guidance technique. The main advantage of the use of ultrasound for this regional anaesthetic technique is a significantly improved success rate compared with landmark-based techniques due to an exact needle positioning. A descriptive study, where punctures were performed by 'fascial click' techniques, illustrates that the tip of the needle position was only correct (i.e. between the internal oblique and transversus abdominis muscles) in 14%, whereas in the remaining 86%, the local anaesthetic was administered in adjacent anatomical structures (ultrasound was used for the confirmation of the tip of the needle). This study may serve as an example for the main reason for failures during landmark-based regional anaesthetic techniques.

The *rectus sheath block* is a useful regional anaesthetic technique in children for umbilical surgery. Our study group developed a technique to achieve rectus sheath blockade with ultrasound. Bilateral (paraumbilical) administration of 0.1mL/kg/side of local anaesthetic in the space between the posterior aspect of the rectus sheath and the rectus abdominis muscle results in successful blocks. An OOP as well as an IP technique can be used for this technique. A poor correlation between the depth of the posterior rectus sheath and weight, height, and body surface area has been found and needs to be recognized.

The *TAP block* can be also used in paediatric patients. The technique is exactly the same as described in adults. The volume of local anaesthetic is recommended as 0.2mL/kg/side with a maximum of 20mL/side.

Suggested further reading

Eichenberger, U., Greher, M., Kirchmair, L., Curatolo, M., Moriggl, B., 2006. Ultrasound-guided blocks of the ilioinguinal and iliohypogastric nerve: accuracy of a selective new technique confirmed by anatomical dissection. *British Journal of Anaesthesia*, 97(2), pp.238–43.

El-Dawlatly, A.A., Turkistani, A., Kettner, S.C., Machata, A.M., Delvi, M.B., Thallaj, A.,Kapral, S., Marhofer, P., (2009). Ultrasound-guided transversus abdominis plane block: description of a new technique and comparison with conventional systemic analgesia during laparoscopic cholecystectomy. *British Journal of Anaesthesia*, 102(6), pp.763–7.

Suresh, S., Chan, V.W., (2009). Ultrasound-guided transversus abdominis plane block in infants, children and adolescents: a simple procedural guidance for their performance. *Pediatric Anesthesia*, 19(4), pp.296–9.

Weintraud, M., Lundblad, M., Kettner, S.C., Willschke, H., Kapral, S., Lönnqvist, P.A., Koppatz, K., Turnheim, K., Bösenberg, A., Marhofer, P., 2009. Ultrasound versus landmark-based technique for ilioinguinal-iliohypogastric nerve blockade in children: the implications on plasma levels of ropivacaine. *Anesthesia & Analgesia*, 108(5), pp.1488–92.

Weintraud, M., Marhofer, P., Bösenberg, A., Kapral, S., Willschke, H., Felfernig, M., Kettner, S., 2008. Ilioinguinal/iliohypogastric blocks in children: where do we administer the local anaesthetic without direct visualization? *Anesthesia & Analgesia*, 106(1), pp.89–93.

Willschke, H., Bösenberg, A., Marhofer, P., Johnston, S., Kettner, S., Eichenberger, U., Wanzel, O., Kapral, S., 2006. Ultrasonographic-guided ilioinguinal/iliohypogastric nerve block in paediatric anaesthesia: what is the optimal volume? *Anesthesia & Analgesia*, 102(6), pp.1680–4.

Willschke, H., Bösenberg, A., Marhofer, P., Johnston, S., Kettner, S., Wanzel, O., Kapral, S., 2006. Ultrasonographic-guided rectus sheath block in paediatric anaesthesia–a new approach to an old technique. *British Journal of Anaesthesia*, 97(2), pp.244–9.

Willschke, H., Marhofer, P., Bösenberg, A., Johnston, S., Wanzel, O., Cox, S., Sitzwohl, C., Kapral, S., 2005. Ultrasonography for ilioinguinal/iliohypogastric nerve blocks in children. *British Journal of Anaesthesia*, 95(2), pp.226–30.

Chapter 16

Neuraxial block techniques

16.1 General considerations

Ultrasonographic-guided neuraxial block techniques in adults are still controversial. The neuronal structures are embedded and protected by bones, cartilages, and massive tendons. All these structures reflect ultrasound beams with subsequent impaired visibility of image qualities. This severe drawback of ultrasound guidance in neuraxial blocks is attenuated in children, where the ossification of the spinal column is incomplete. Thus, epidural blockade (single shot or catheter placement) under ultrasound assistance is well investigated and established in children, but associated with significant problems in adults.

Considering the technical troubles with epidural ultrasound in adults, the paravertebral approach as a (mainly) unilateral regional anaesthetic technique seems to be an excellent option. The entire topic of paravertebral ultrasound is currently under intensive investigation and the technique described below is based on the current knowledge regarding this topic.

16.2 Epidural blocks

16.2.1 Anatomy

The spine is composed of 7 cervical, 12 thoracic, and 5 lumbar vertebrae as well as sacral and coccygeal portions (Figure 16.1). Despite described cervical approaches to the epidural space, only the thoracic and lumbar approaches are of practical interest.

The following osseous components are integral parts of the vertebrae:

- *Corpus vertebrae*: cylindrical in shape, connected by the intervertebral discs, front side convex, back side concave.
- *Pedicles*: two short and thick processes, projecting backwards from the upper part of the body at the junction of the posterior and lateral surfaces, concavities above and below pedicles are named vertebral notches and form the intervertebral foramina.

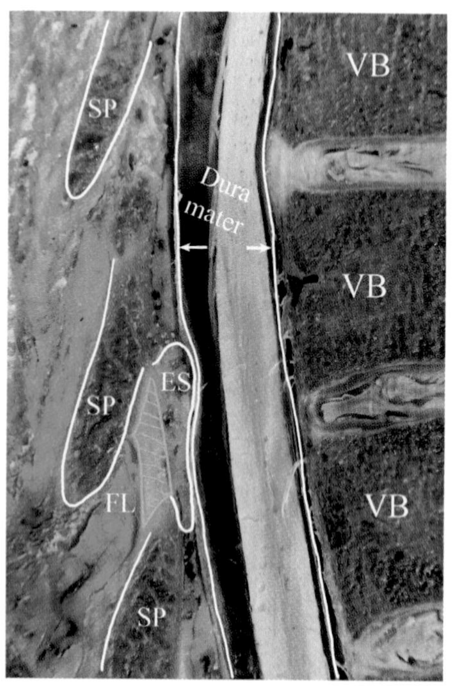

Fig. 16.1 Anatomical longitudinal view of the lower thoracic part of the spine. SP: spinous process; FL: flavum ligament; ES: epidural space; VB: vertebral body.

- *Laminae*: two broad plates directed backwards and medially from the pedicles, fuse in the posterior midline to complete the posterior boundary of the vertebral foramen, ligamenta flava attach to upper borders and lower parts of the anterior surfaces.
- *Spinous processes*: directed backwards and downwards from the junction of the laminae, overlapping at thoracic levels, more horizontal at lumbar levels, muscles and ligaments attach at spinous processes.
- *Articular processes*: two superior and two inferior from the junctions of the pedicles and laminae, coated with hyaline cartilage.
- *Transverse processes*: one on either side from the point where the laminae join the pedicles (between the superior and inferior articular processes), muscles and ligaments attach at transverse processes.

The vertebral bodies are connected with the following ligaments:

- *Supraspinal ligament*: a strong fibrous cord between the apices of the spinous processes.
- *Interspinal ligament*: thin and membranous, connect adjacent spinous processes, extend from the root to apex of each process, narrow and elongated in the thoracic region, broader in the lumbar region.

- *Flavum ligament*: inserts inferiorly onto the superior edge and the postero-superior surface of the caudal lamina and superiorly to the inferior edge and antero-inferior surface of the cephalad lamina, composed of a 2.5–3.5mm thick superficial and 1mm thin deep component.
- *Posterior longitudinal ligament*: within the vertebral canal, extends along the posterior surfaces of the vertebral bodies.
- *Anterior longitudinal ligament*: extends along the anterior surfaces of the vertebral bodies.

The following meningeal structures cover the spinal medulla:

- *Dura mater:* forms a loose sheath around the spinal medulla, separated from the arachnoidea by the subdural cavity, separated from the wall of the vertebral canal by the *epidural space* (contains a quantity of loose areolar tissue and venous plexuses).
- *Arachnoidea:* thin membrane, separated from the dura by the *subdural space* (contains a quantity of loose areolar tissue and venous plexuses), surrounds the spinal nerves.
- *Pia mater:* covers the entire surface of the spinal medulla, is adherent to it, form sheaths to spinal nerves.

16.2.2 Ultrasound-guided technique

A lower frequency sector probe should be used for neuraxial ultrasound in adults. The best visibility of the neuraxial structures can be obtained with a longitudinal, paramedian probe position. Depending on the individual ultrasound windows, the dura mater and spinal cord can be visualized. The spinous processes and laminae cause significant shadows, thus decreasing the overall visibility of the neuraxial structures. The flavum ligament is difficult to visualize to due its anisotropy. Calcification of the supra- and interspinal ligaments may also impair the visibility to the neuraxial structures, particular in the elderly. Due to the different angulations of the spinous processes (see Section 16.2.1), ultrasound visualization of the lumbar neuraxial structures should be less impaired compared with thoracic parts.

16.2.3 Practical block technique

With the patient in a sitting or lateral position and a kyphotic formed (flexed) spine, the sector probe should be positioned in a longitudinal, paramedian manner. Following this probe position, parts of the dura mater and the spinal cord can be visualized (Figure 16.2). It is important to state that in many cases, an adequate visualization of the relevant neuraxial structures is impossible, which depends on the individual grade of formation of shades caused by osseous structures and calcification of ligaments. The epidural space can be

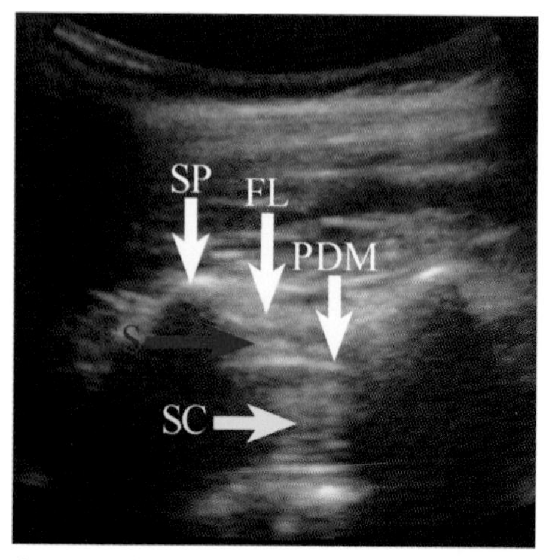

Fig. 16.2 Ultrasound image of the epidural space at the lower part of the spine. ES: epidural space; SP: spinous process; FL: flavum ligament; PDM: posterior dura mater; SC: spinal cord; left side=cranial.

identified as a slightly hyperechoic space posterior to the dura mater. Vessels may be identifiable by Doppler ultrasound.

An IP needle guidance technique should be used with a medial approach of the cannula to the epidural space (Figure 16.3). The practical block technique is always a combination of the traditional loss-of-resistance (LOR) and ultrasound guidance. The main sign of a correct epidural position of the needle tip is the downward movement of the dura mater, which should be confirmed

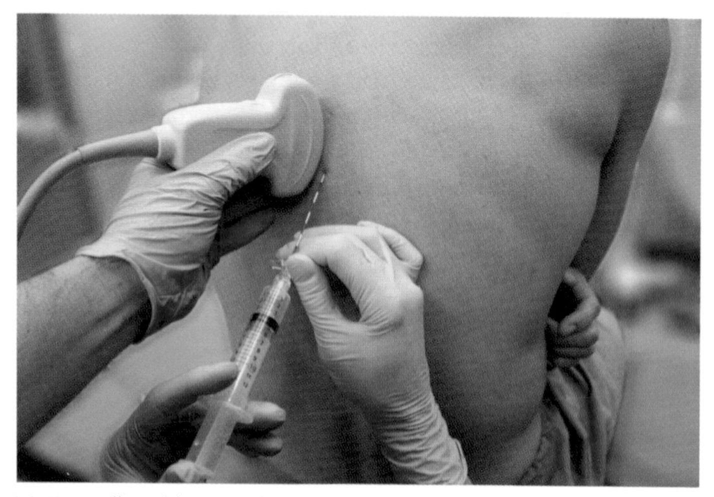

Fig. 16.3 IP needle guidance technique for optimal visualization of the neuraxial structures during adult epidural blockade.

after a successful LOR and, in cases of an epidural catheter placement, via the administration of the local anaesthetic through the epidural catheter. The local anaesthetic appears hypoechoic inside the epidural space. Accordingly, care should be taken to avoid the injection of air bubbles during LOR and the administration of local anaesthetic through the epidural catheter.

16.2.4 Essentials

Block characteristic	Advanced technique
Patient position	Sitting or lateral with flexed spine
Ultrasound equipment	2–5MHz sector probe
Specific ultrasound setting	Low to medium frequencies
Important anatomical structures	Dura mater
Ultrasound appearance of the neuronal structures	The spinal cord appear as longitudinal, parallel structure
Needle equipment	Tuohy needle (18G in most cases)
Needle guidance technique	IP with a medial needle position and longitudinal, paramedian probe position
Estimated local anaesthetic volume	Dependent on the specific demands of the epidural blockade (between 8–15mL)

16.3 Paravertebral blocks

16.3.1 Anatomy

The thoracic paravertebral space (TPVS) is located bilaterally to the vertebral column and defined as a wedge-shaped space. The anterolateral boundary is formed by the parietal pleura, the medial boundary is built by the posterolateral aspect of the vertebral body, the intervertebral disc, the intervertebral foramen and its contents, and the internal intercostal membrance (IIM) with its medical continuation, the superior costotransverse ligament which extends from the lower border of the transverse process above to the upper border of the transverse process below forms the posterior wall of the paravertebral space. The apex of the paravertebral space is continuous with the intercostal space lateral to the tips of the transverse processes. The endothoracic fascia, which is interposed between the parietal pleura and the superior costotransverse ligament, divides the paravertebral space in two compartments, the anterior extrapleural and the posterior subendothoracic paravertebral compartment. The TPVS contains the intercostal spinal nerves, dorsal rami, rami communicantes, the sympathetic chain, intercostal vessels, and fatty tissue. The intercostal nerve and vessels are located behind the endothoracic fascia while the sympathetic trunk is located anterior to it in the paravertebral space (Figure 16.4).

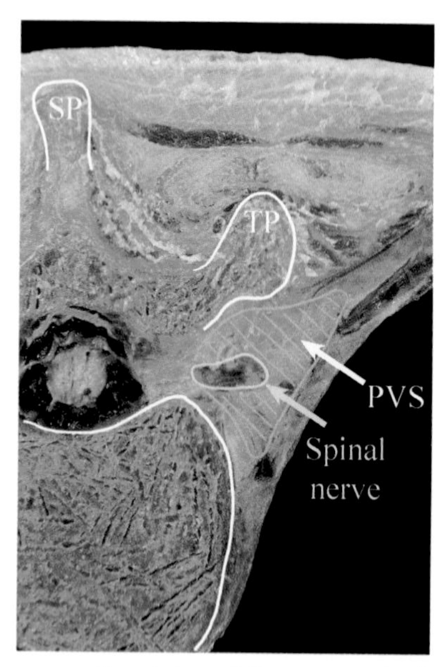

Fig. 16.4 Anatomical cross-sectional view of the paravertebral space. PVS: paravertebral space; SP: spinous process; TP: transverse process; left side=medial.

16.3.2 Ultrasound-guided technique

We recommend a lateral approach to the paravertebral space with the IIM as main guidance structure. A 38–45mm linear probe is appropriate to visualize the IIM. Starting with a scanning head position from the midline, the probe should be moved laterally until the transverse process in visualized. A slightly oblique probe position is usually required to identify the IIM (Figures 16.5 and 16.6).

16.3.3 Practical block technique

Once the transverse process, the IIM, and the parietal pleura are adequately visualized, an OOP needle guidance technique should be performed as illustrated in Figure 16.5 with the patient in a sitting position and with a flexed spine. In principle, an IP needle guidance technique from the lateral can also be considered, but this technique is more difficult since the distance between the puncture point and the target is significantly longer compared with the OOP technique. The rotated position of the probe also makes the IP needle guidance technique more difficult.

The tip of the needle should be visualized after piercing the IIM. Care is required to avoid damage of the pleura. After aspiration to avoid an inadvertent

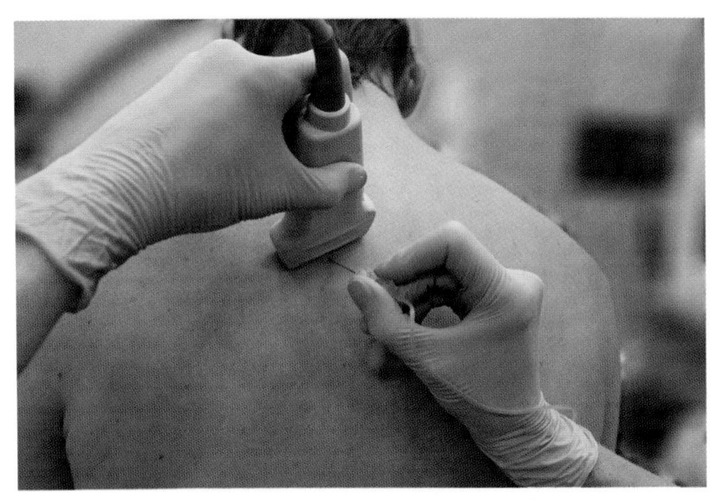

Fig. 16.5 Scanning head position for optimal visualization of the paravertebral space and OOP needle guidance technique.

intravascular position of the tip of the needle, the local anaesthetic can be administered. Downward movement of the pleura is an optimal sign of the correct placement of the local anaesthetic (Figure 16.7). The haemodynamics should be carefully observed during and after the blockade since an effective sympatholysis may cause bradycardia and hypotension.

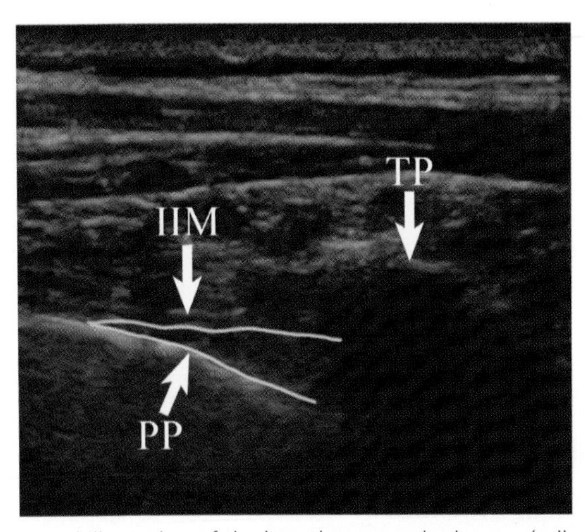

Fig. 16.6 Ultrasound illustration of the lateral paravertebral space (yellow lines) between the IIM, the transverse process, and the parietal pleura. IIM: internal intercostal membrane; TP: transverse process; PP: parietal pleura; left side=lateral.

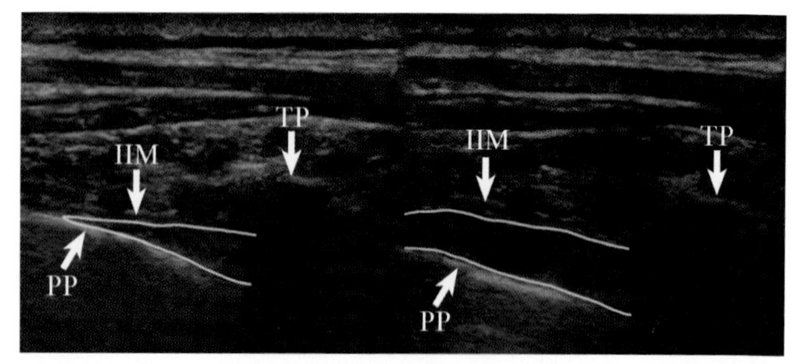

Fig. 16.7 The paravertebral space is clearly identified on the left side of the illustration between the internal intercostal membrance, the transverse process, and the parietal pleura. Following administration of 15mL of local anaesthetic, the paravertebral space is opened and the pleura is moved downwards. IIM: internal intercostal membrane; TP: transverse process; PP: parietal pleura; left side=lateral.

Depending on the required analgesia, punctures at two different levels are useful. It seems that paravertebral catheters are ineffective to achieve a spacious spread of local anaesthetic by using a lateral approach. Future investigations will show if catheter placement is facilitated with a more medial approach.

16.3.4 **Essentials**

Block characteristic	Advanced technique
Patient position	Sitting or lateral with flexed spine
Ultrasound equipment	38–50mm linear probe
Specific ultrasound setting	Medium frequencies
Important anatomical structures	Transverse process, internal intercostal membrane, parietal pleura
Ultrasound appearance of the neuronal structures	In most cases, the neuronal structures are not visible (isoechoic)
Needle equipment	70mm, Facette tip
Needle guidance technique	OOP
Estimated local anaesthetic volume	10–15mL/injection, a maximum of two injections should be performed

16.4 **Implications in children**

16.4.1 **Epidural blockade**

Ultrasound guidance during epidural catheter placement increases its safety because of the direct visualization of neuraxial structures, which is

Table 8 Neuraxial visibility by ultrasound in different age groups

Age (mths)	Weight (kg)	% Dura visibility		Overall visibility (V0–3)		Acoustic shadows (S0–3)	
		Lumbar	Thoracic	Lumbar	Thoracic	Lumbar	Thoracic
0–3	4.1 ± 1.3	80 ± 14	70 ± 32	2.9 ± 0.3	2.4 ± 0.7	2.2 ± 0.4	2.1 ± 0.8
4–14	10.9 ± 2.5	58 ± 15	28 ± 13	2.6 ± 0.6	1.2 ± 0.4	1.8 ± 0.4	1.2 ± 0.4
15–35	14.0 ± 2.0	41 ± 13	29 ± 13	2.1 ± 0.4	1.4 ± 0.5	1.6 ± 0.5	1.1 ± 0.4
36–94	19.7 ± 2.8	30 ± 17	21 ± 13	1.7 ± 0.8	1.5 ± 0.7	1.5 ± 0.5	1.1 ± 0.5

V0=not visible, V1=somewhat visible, V2=reasonable visible, V3=fully visible.
S0=fully shadowed, S1=major shadows, S2=minor shadows, S3=no shadows.

optimal in neonates and infants and decreases in older children (Table 8). The longitudinal paramedian approach provides the best visualization of the dura mater, which is the *main guidance structure* during the performance of epidurals (Figure 16.8). The most recommended technique is a combination of ultrasound guidance and the traditional LOR method (Figure 16.9), and the correct spread of local anaesthetic inside the epidural space is identified by a downward movement of the dura mater (Figure 16.10). Identification of the catheter is possible in most cases by using the maximum frequency of the ultrasound probe (Figure 16.11). Identification of the position of the epidural catheter is also possible in a cross-sectional view (Figure 16.12).

The appropriate size of the needle equipment is mandatory for a successful performance of epidurals in children. Needle manufacturers have designed 21G Tuohy needles and 25G catheters with wire, but these catheters tend to kink and therefore, larger needle and catheters sizes are more appropriate for continuous techniques. In small weight groups, the epidural space must be

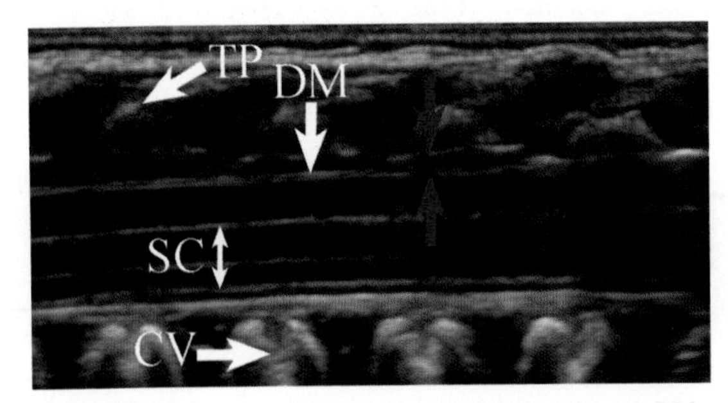

Fig. 16.8 Ultrasound illustration of the neuraxial structures in a 1,500g neonate. TP: transverse process; DM: dura mater; SC: spinal cord; CV: corpus vertebrae; left side=cranial. The blue arrows indicate the epidural space.

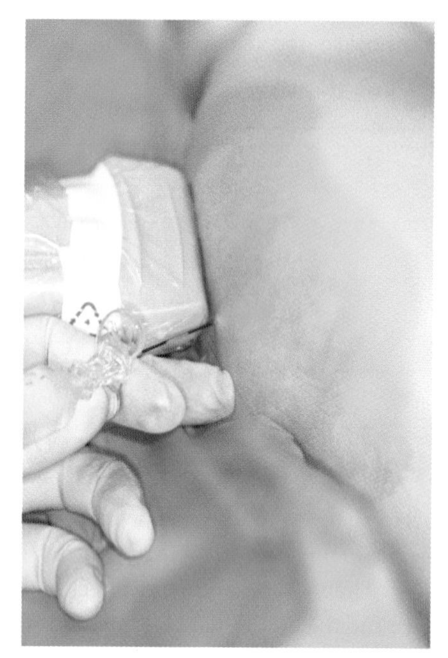

Fig. 16.9 Position of the needle relative to the ultrasound probe for epidural puncture with the patient in a lateral position.

widened by an initial injection of fluid (we use local anaesthetic for the LOR to avoid dilution of the local anaesthetic by other fluids with resulting unknown final anaesthetic concentration) to facilitate catheter placement. Therefore, a 24G or even 22G catheter can be pushed forward usually without problems and the subsequent advantage of minimizing the risk of catheter kinking.

Especially in small weight groups, it is difficult to keep the volumes of local anaesthetics as suggested in the 'Essentials'. Usually more local anaesthetic will be administered by the LOR technique and the further ultrasound confirmation of the correct placement of the catheter also needs the administration of

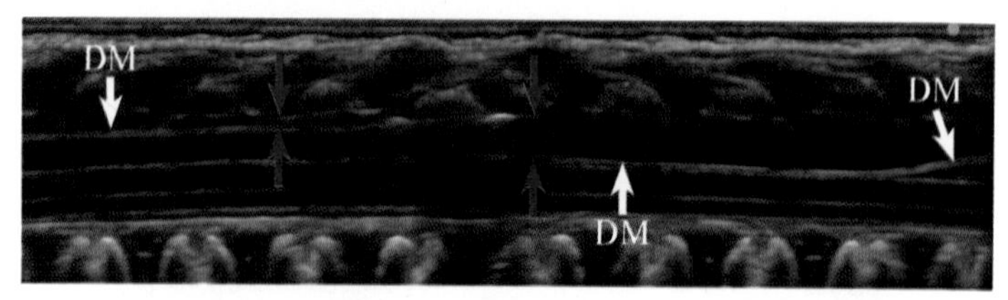

Fig. 16.10 Downward movement of the dura mater (DM) in a 1,500g neonate after the administration of local anaesthetic (left side of image). The blue arrows indicate the epidural space before (left side of image) and after the administration of local anaesthetic (right side of image).

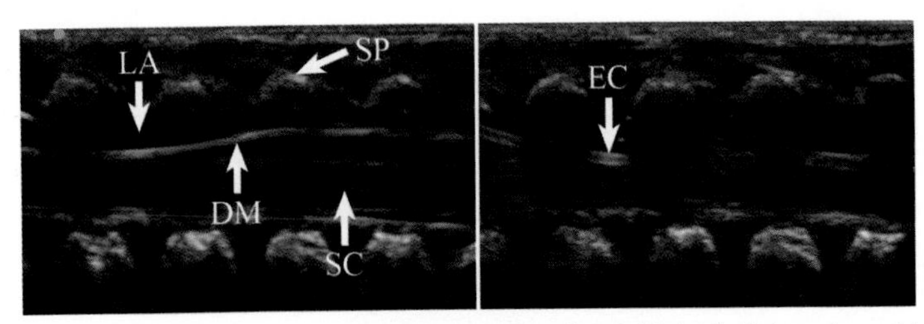

Fig. 16.11 Identification of the epidural catheter after initial administration of local anaesthetic to open the epidural space. EC: epidural catheter; LA: local anaesthetic; SP: spinous process; DM: dura mater; SC: spinal cord; left side in both images=cranial.

local anaesthetics. Children's haemodynamics are relatively inert to high sympathetic blocks; in fact, we have never observed such haemodynamic-related side effects in our clinical practice. It is still a matter of ongoing discussion if the subsequent management of the epidural catheter should be based on a continuous infusion or a bolus administration. We tend to use more and more the bolus administration (twice a day) with a low concentration of local anaesthetic to reduce the overall drug exposure and to provide an adequate spread of the block.

16.4.1.2 Essentials

Block characteristic	Intermediate technique
Patient position	Lateral
Ultrasound equipment	25–38mm linear probe
Specific ultrasound setting	Highest frequencies
Important anatomical structures	Dura mater, subarachnoid space, spinal cord
Ultrasound appearance of the neuronal structures	Hyperechoic
Needle equipment	<1,000g: 21G Tuohy needle, 25G catheter 1–4kg: 20G Tuohy needle, 24G catheter 4–25kg: 19G Tuohy needle, 22G catheter>25kg: 18G Tuohy needle, 20G catheter
Needle guidance technique	IP with medial needle position and paramedian longitudinal probe position
Estimated local anaesthetic volume	About 0.4mL/kg for thoracic approaches About 0.5mL/kg for lumbar approaches

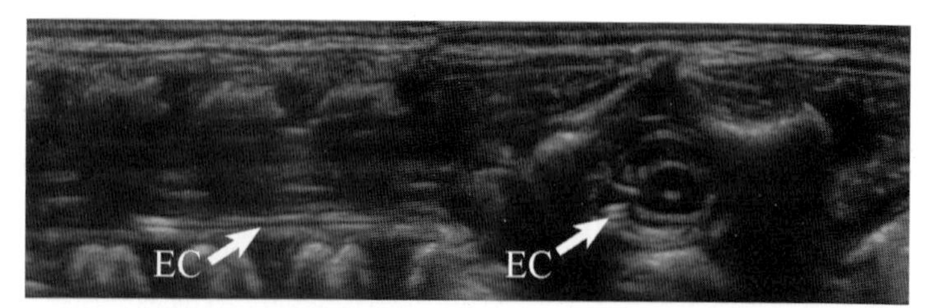

Fig. 16.12 Longitudinal (left side of image) and cross-sectional (right side of image) views of an epidural catheter (EC) in a 1,900g neonate. The catheter is in an anterior position.

16.4.2 Caudal blockade

Ultrasound visualization of the spread of local anaesthetic can also be used for caudal blockade, which is the most popular, regional anaesthetic technique in children. The caudal puncture itself is easy to perform because of the clear anatomical landmarks (sacrococcygeal membrane and sacral hiatus) and it seems obvious to us that the observation of the correct spread of local anaesthetic should be associated with an increased safety and effectiveness (Figures 16.13 and 16.14). Ultrasound can also be used in cases of technical difficulties to puncture the sacrococcygeal membrane by direct visualization of the sacral hiatus and the membrane itself (Figure 16.15).

16.4.2.1 Essentials

Block characteristic	Basic technique
Patient position	Lateral
Ultrasound equipment	38mm linear probe
Specific ultrasound setting	High frequencies
Important anatomical structures	Dura mater
Ultrasound appearance of the neuronal structures	Hyperechoic
Needle equipment	24G, 45°
Needle guidance technique	IP with medial needle position and paramedian longitudinal probe position
Estimated local anaesthetic volume	1mL/kg

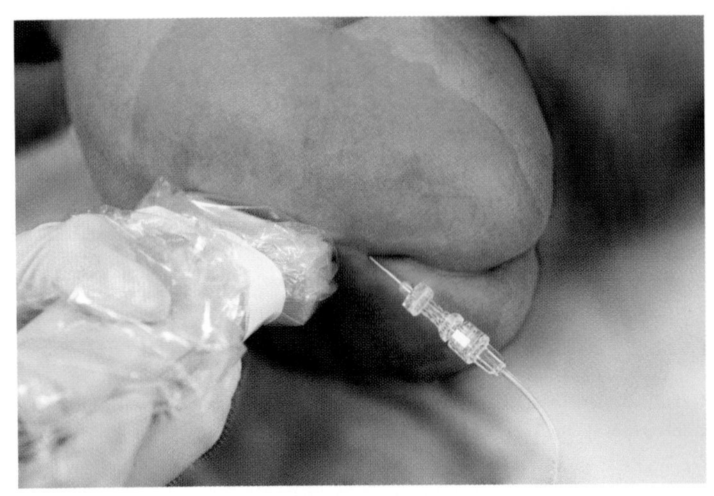

Fig. 16.13 Position of the ultrasound probe during caudal blockade in a 3kg baby.

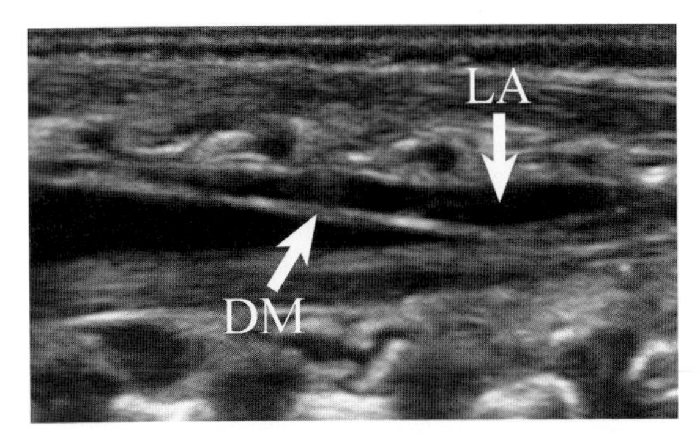

Fig. 16.14 The spread of local anaesthetic can be visualized clearly during injection where the dura mater moves downward (in the ultrasound illustration) during injection of the local anaesthetic. LA: local anaesthetic; DM: dura mater; left side=cranial.

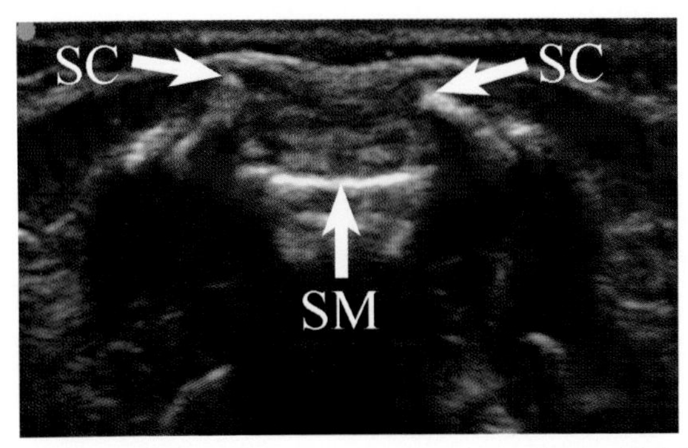

Fig. 16.15 Cross-sectional view of the sacrococcygeal membrane (SM) between the sacral cornuae (SC).

Suggested further reading

Karmakar, M.K., 2001. Thoracic paravertebral block. *Anaesthesiology*, 95(3), pp.771–80.

Karmakar, M.K., Ho, A.M., Li, X., Kwok, W.H., Tsang, K., Ngan Kee, W.D., 2008. Ultrasound-guided lumbar plexus block through the acoustic window of the lumbar ultrasound trident. *British Journal of Anaesthesia*, 100(4), pp.533–7.

Karmakar, M.K., Li, X., Ho, A.M., Kwok, W.H., Chui, P.T., 2009. Real-time ultrasound-guided paramedian epidural access: evaluation of a novel in-plane technique. *British Journal of Anaesthesia*, 102(6), pp.845–54.

Luyet, C., Eichenberger, U., Greif, R., Vogt, A., Szücs Farkas, Z., Moriggl, B., 2009. Ultrasound-guided paravertebral puncture and placement of catheters in human cadavers: an imaging study. *British Journal of Anaesthesia*, 102(4), pp.534–9.

Marhofer, P., Bösenberg, A., Sitzwohl, C., Willschke, H., Wanzel, O., Kapral, S., 2005. Pilot study of neuraxial imaging by ultrasound in infants and children. *Pediatric Anesthesia*, 15(8), pp.671–6.

Marhofer, P., Kettner, S.C., Hajbok, L., Dubsky, P., Fleischmann, E., 2010. Lateral ultrasound-guided paravertebral blockade: an anatomical-based description of a new technique. *British Journal of Anaesthesia*, Advance Access published August 3rd 2010.

Richardson, J., Lönnqvist, P.A., 1998. Thoracic paravertebral block. *British Journal of Anaesthesia*, 81(2), pp.230–8.

Willschke, H., Bosenberg, A., Marhofer, P., Willschke, J., Schwindt, J., Weintraud, M., Kapral, S., Kettner, S., 2007. Epidural catheter placement in neonates: sonoanatomy and feasibility of ultrasonographic guidance in term and preterm neonates. *Regional Anesthesia and Pain Medicine*, 32(1), pp.34–40.

Willschke, H., Marhofer, P., Bösenberg, A., Johnston, S., Wanzel, O., Sitzwohl, C., Kettner, S., Kapral, S., 2006. Epidural catheter placement in children: comparing a novel approach using ultrasound guidance and a standard loss-of-resistance technique. *British Journal of Anaesthesia*, 97(2), pp.200–7.

Chapter 17

Peripheral catheter techniques

Recent developments in perineural catheter technology deal with the topic of ultrasound and continuous regional blocks. We are at the beginning of an evolution and the entire topic needs an exact scientific evaluation. This very short chapter highlights the theoretical considerations and the author's personal experience.

All relevant blocks could be performed as single blocks, but also as continuous techniques. Facette tip and Tuohy needles can be used as introduction cannulas where the catheter can be advanced. According to the particular tip of the introduction cannula, the catheter will be advanced along the course of the needle (Figure 17.1) or will deviate from it (Figure 17.2).

The technique itself to visualize the neuronal structures is equal. During positioning of the catheter, it could be directly visualized in most cases (Figure 17.3), but more importantly, the spread of local anaesthetic can be observed. We suggest for the fixation of a peripheral nerve block catheter an adhesive and transparent tape where daily ultrasonographic investigation of the spread of local anaesthetic is possible.

By using ultrasound for the detection of the spread of local anaesthetic, important information has been acquired regarding the block mechanism of specific approaches. Despite a lack of scientific studies in this field, an initial evaluation of meaningful catheter approaches could be performed. Due to the fact that ultrasound-guided regional block techniques are strictly performed by multi-injections, clear recommendations in this field could be provided.

The following peripheral techniques can be recommended for a continuous blockade:

- Interscalene.
- Supraclavicular.
- Femoral.
- Sciatic (subgluteal and mid-femoral approaches).

Future scientific studies have to evaluate the usefulness and practicability of ultrasound-guided perineural catheters.

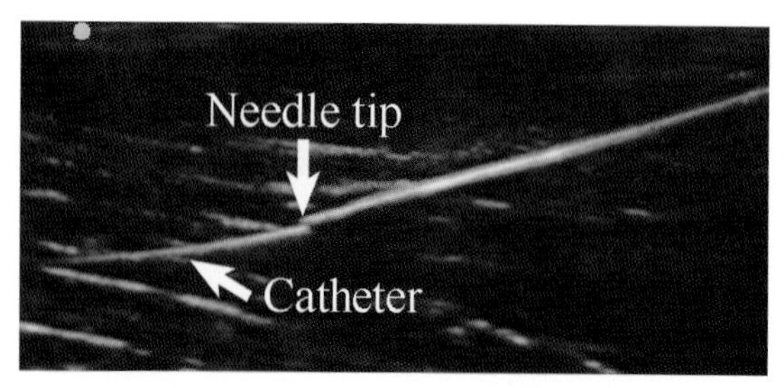

Fig. 17.1 Advancement of a catheter through a Facette tip needle.

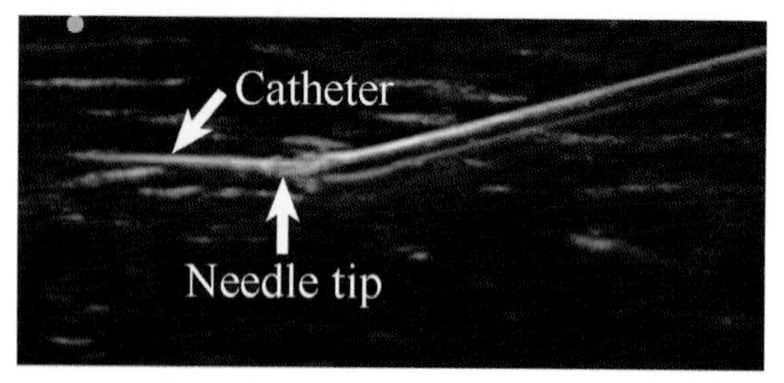

Fig. 17.2 Advancement of a catheter through a Tuohy tip needle.

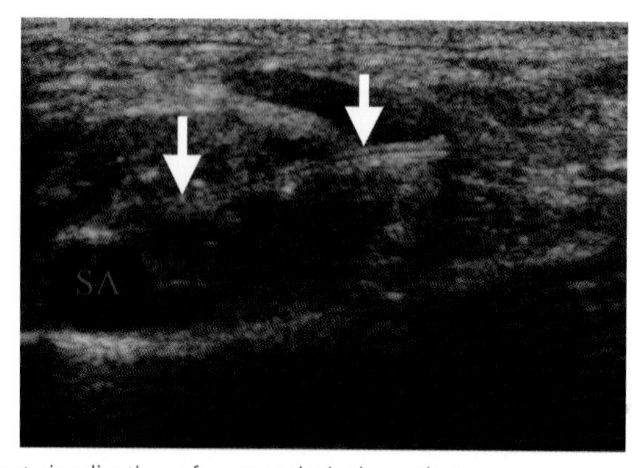

Fig. 17.3 Direct visualization of a supraclavicular catheter.

Suggested further reading

Koscielniak–Nielsen, Z.J., Rasmussen, H., Hesselbjerg, L., 2008. Long-axis ultrasound imaging of the nerves and advancement of perineural catheters under direct vision: a preliminary report of four cases. *Regional Anesthesia and Pain Medicine*, 33(5), pp.477–82.

Chapter 18

Future perspectives

18.1 Regional blocks for particular patient populations

Ultrasound-guided regional anaesthetic techniques in particular patient populations are currently not being investigated. In daily clinical practice, we are more and more confronted with obese patients or with those who have significant diseases. In particular, obesity is a rapidly growing pandemic phenomenon (Table 9) and therefore, scientific efforts have to focus on this highly clinically relevant problem.

Other patient populations that may benefit from regional anaesthesia are the extremely old and young patients. During the past years, a lot has been published regarding paediatric regional anaesthesia, but regional anaesthesia in the elderly still focuses on neuraxial techniques. But it is a matter of fact that in the next decades, the population will become older and older and therefore, the number of patients over 80 years old will increase significantly. Thus, scientific and clinical efforts also have to focus on these patients.

18.2 Education

Currently, learning tools, education, and certification in the use of ultrasonography in regional anaesthesia are under intensive discussion. Chapter 4 mentions education and adequate training as a non-technical limitation. In fact, the quality of education and training will be one of the most important factors in the overall development of ultrasound-guided regional anaesthesia. It is a consensus that new learning tools are required to improve teaching in this fast-growing field of anaesthesia. Most of the traditional textbooks already include chapters on ultrasound-guided nerve blocks. New textbooks with a focus on ultrasound-guided nerve blocks are available. The authors of this text sincerely hope that their practical and scientific experience of more than 15 years in ultrasonography in regional anaesthesia support the worldwide enthusiasm in that field.

Modern learning tools, such as interactive DVDs, are also available. Not available is an anatomy textbook fulfilling the needs of the anaesthetist who is interested in ultrasound anatomy. Cross-sectional anatomy is needed for

Table 9 Increase in prevalence (%) of overweight (BMI ≥25), obesity (BMI ≥30), and severe obesity (BMI ≥40) among US adults*

	Overweight	**Obese**	**Severely obese**
1999–2000	64.5	30.5	4.7
1988–1994	56.0	23.0	2.9
1976–1980	46.0	14.4	No data

* Source: CDC, National Center for Health Statistics, National Health and Nutrition Examination Survey. Health, United States, 2002.

ultrasound guidance in regional anaesthesia. More specifically, irregular cross-sectional views are used in most cases in order to visualize the targeted nerve perpendicularly. Furthermore, anatomic descriptions of the adjacent structures of nerves, with a clear focus on possible damages by the advancing needle, are needed. The descriptions should include ultrasound images with marked anatomic structures to enable analyses of these images. This current book tries to obey this highly sophisticated concept.

In contrast to the learning tool, certification in the use of ultrasonography in regional anaesthesia is under controversy. Some anaesthetists suggest a certification similar to the examinations in transoesophageal echocardiography. However, the introduction of mandatory examinations might improve the quality, but might hinder the promotion of the technique. Therefore, we have to bear in mind that potentially more dangerous techniques of indirect needle guidance are performed without any additional examinations. A compromise might be a defined training for instructors similar to the training in advanced life support. Figure 4.3 provides a suggestion for a concept in training in ultrasound-guided regional anaesthesia.

18.3 **Technical developments**

Ultrasonography has not been developed as a guidance technique for regional anaesthesia. In fact, inventive anaesthetists have used the existing technique for their needs. Ultrasound has a number of specific advantages. One of the greatest advantages of ultrasound in regional anaesthesia is that fluids are extremely well visualized because of their hypoechoic appearance. Equally, the spread of local anaesthetic in human tissues is easy to visualize. However, there are also specific problems which might hinder the use of ultrasonography in daily clinical practice of regional anaesthesia. A major drawback of ultrasonography is that the ultrasound beam is extremely narrow. Therefore, the inexperienced user will regularly lose visualization of the needle while performing a nerve block. Even minimal changes of the position of the ultrasound probe result in loss of needle visibility. A possible solution to this problem would be the use of real-time, three-dimensional ultrasound probes (4D). Such probes are already available and are currently used in echocardiography and obstetrics. Matrix-array ultrasound produces real-time 3D images by using a square array of transducers to steer the ultrasound beam in three dimensions electronically with no moving parts. However, the available 3D probes are not useful for ultrasound guidance in regional anaesthesia due to certain technical limitations. Firstly, the transducers in a regular two-dimensional (2D) ultrasound probe have a linear array, and to reach a lateral resolution adequate for the visualization of small structures such as nerves, modern ultrasound probes carry 256 parallel transducers. 3D ultrasound probes carry 64 times 64 transducers and therefore, have a reduced lateral resolution. Secondly, the axial resolution of 3D probes is also a problem. These probes are used for relatively deep structures such as a beating heart or a foetus. Therefore, their frequency with approximately 4.5MHz is relatively low, giving a lateral resolution not suitable for most regional anaesthetic techniques. Other medical applications such as ultrasound-guided breast biopsy are faced with the problem of needle guidance. The development of 3D ultrasound-guided breast biopsy systems is already advanced. High resolution, real-time, three-dimensional ultrasonography (4D) will probably be available in the next ten years. This future technique will facilitate ultrasound guidance in regional anaesthesia dramatically. Furthermore, it has the potential to reduce the complication rates of regional anaesthesia further due to the improved visibility of the needle while advancing it through tissue close to the aimed nerve structure. From today's point of view, our main focus should be on optimizing our skills with 2D ultrasound.

Appendix 1

Zuers Ultrasound Experts regional anaesthesia statement

Participants (in alphabetic order)

Vincent Chan
Department of Anaesthesia and Pain Management,
University Health Network,
Toronto Western Hospital,
Toronto, Ontario, Canada

Manfred Greher
Department of Anaesthesiology,
Perioperative Intensive Care and Pain Therapy,
Herz-Jesu Hospital,
Vienna, Austria

Markus Hollmann
Academic Medical Centre,
Department of Anaesthesia,
University of Amsterdam,
Amsterdam, The Netherlands

Stephan Kapral
Department of Anaesthesia,
General Intensive Care and Pain Control,
Medical University of Vienna,
Vienna, Austria

Stephan Kettner
Department of Anaesthesia,
General Intensive Care and Pain Control,
Medical University of Vienna,
Vienna, Austria

Zbigniew Koscielniak–Nielsen
Department of Anaesthesia and Operative Services,
Rigshospital,
Copenhagen, Denmark

Per–Arne Lönnqvist
Paediatric Anaesthesia & Intensive Care,
Astrid Lindgrens Children's Hospital,
Karolinska University Hospital,
Stockholm, Sweden

David MacLeod
Division of Orthopaedics,
Plastics & Regional Anaesthesia,
Department of Anaesthesiology,
Duke University Medical Centre,
Durham, North Carolina, USA

Peter Marhofer
Department of Anaesthesia,
General Intensive Care and Pain Control,
Medical University of Vienna,
Vienna, Austria

Colin McCartney
Department of Anaesthesia,
Sunnybrook Health Sciences Centre,
Toronto, Ontario, Canada

Barry Nicholls
Taunton & Somerset NHS Trust
Musgrove Park Hospital,
Taunton, Somerset, United Kingdom

Yukata Satoh
Department of Anaesthesia,
Goshogawara Municipal Hospital,
Goshogawara City, Aomori, Japan

Robert Weller
Department of Anaesthesiology,
Wake Forest University School of Medicine,
Medical Centre Blvd,
Winston-Salem, North Carolina, USA

Harald Willschke
Medical University of Vienna,
Department of Anaesthesia,
General Intensive Care and Pain Control,
Medical University of Vienna,
Vienna, Austria

Preamble

During the past ten years, ultrasound guidance for regional anaesthetic techniques has shown increasing popularity. Techniques for placing local anaesthetic adjacent to nerve structures have become more consistent with the use of ultrasound guidance and the technology has been adopted by anaesthetists around the world. Despite this, there is little consistency and few recommendations as to what constitutes the best method to describe, perform, and teach many of these techniques. This could potentially hinder rather than promote the use of this valuable new technology, especially for new users.

A meeting of 14 experts from eight different countries and three continents with a combined experience of many thousand ultrasound-guided blocks was held in Zuers, Austria from January 7th to 12th in 2007 to consider recommendations to promote consistency in both the teaching and practice of ultrasound-guided regional anaesthesia. It was the aim of the group to promote the use of ultrasound by describing guidelines to facilitate the performance of ultrasound-guided, single-injection techniques in adults for regional anaesthesia and acute pain control. This encompassed recommendations for the safe performance, grading of block performance difficulty, and standardization of nomenclature for nerve visualization, and teaching recommendations. It was also recognized by the group that the evidence base for the use of these techniques is developing and therefore, some of these recommendations may be revised in the future, depending on further studies as they become available. These recommendations therefore represent the opinion of a group of highly experienced practitioners and it is hoped that the recommendations may be of use to practitioners who are either starting to learn ultrasound-guided regional techniques or who wish to improve their existing techniques.

The group did not consider the use of ultrasound for regional anaesthesia in children or for guidance of interventional pain procedures. This may be the subject of future recommendations.

Decision process

- Stage 1: Selection of expert panel based on one or more of the following criteria—Medline review, experience in education, significant clinical experience with ultrasound, special knowledge in regional anaesthesia.
- Stage 2: Identification of preliminary areas of importance in the field of ultrasonography in regional anaesthesia based on a survey carried out one month prior to the expert meeting.

- Stage 3: Meeting in Zuers, Austria, Europe from January 7th to 12th, 2007.
- Stage 4: Post-meeting questionnaire of 'Ultrasound-guided Nerve Block Rating Scale'.
- Stage 5: Analysis of results and a 3-month email-based discussion following the completion of the first draft of the expert statement.
- Stage 6: Final expert meeting statement.

Recommendations for the appropriate, safe, and effective performance of ultrasound-guided techniques

- Start with basic block techniques.
- Use a machine and transducer capable of the highest resolution imaging at the target depth.
- Optimize machine settings to visualize the nerve(s) whenever possible.
- Orientate the transducer perpendicular (90°) to the anatomical course of the target structure(s) for optimal visualization.
- Maintain continuous awareness of the needle tip location.
- Choose a needle path that allows proximity of the needle tip to the nerve without needle-nerve contact.
- Immobile needle technique is suggested to allow careful maintenance of needle tip position during injection.
- Visualize the spread of local anaesthetic during injection. If no spread is visible, consider that intravascular injection may have occurred.
- Achieve circumferential spread of local anaesthetic where a discrete single nerve is visible. Limit further injection once circumneural spread is accomplished.
- Consider the use of a nerve stimulator to confirm the nerve identity and to reduce the risk of intraneural injection if the target nerve structure is not clearly seen.

Definitions

Currently, various definitions of the 'position of the needle relative to the nerve' and the 'needle relative to the probe' are used. A uniform definition of the 'position of the needle relative to the nerve' and the 'needle relative to the probe' facilitates the understanding of future discussions and publications in the field of 'ultrasonographic-guided regional blocks'.

Needle relative to the nerve

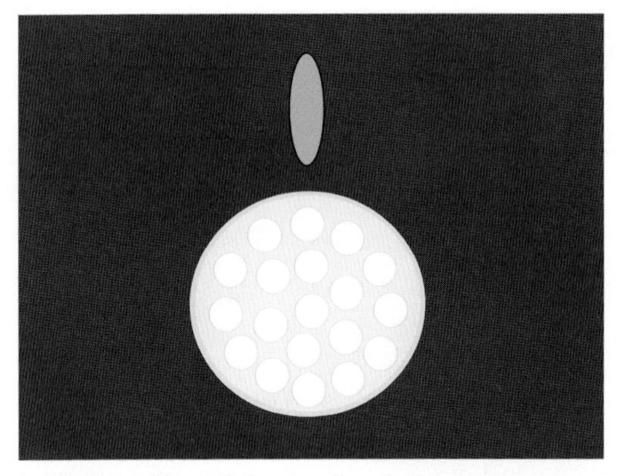

Fig. A1 Short axis (SAX) position of the needle relative to the nerve.

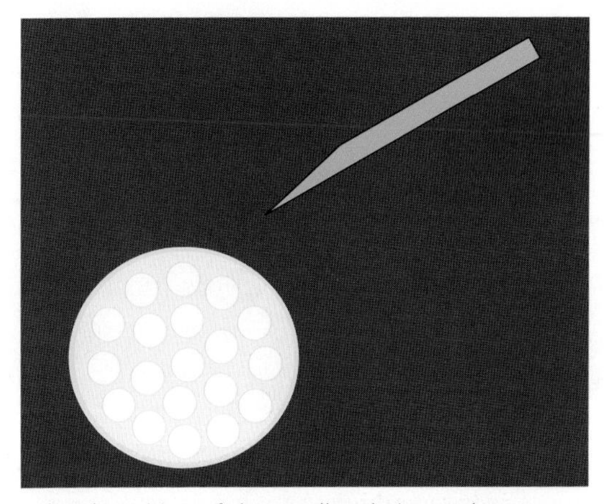

Fig. A2 Long axis (LAX) position of the needle relative to the nerve.

Needle relative to the probe

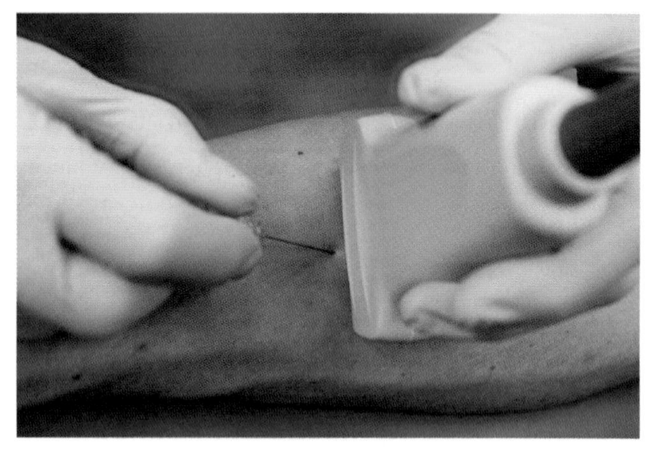

Fig. A3 OOP position of the needle relative to the probe.

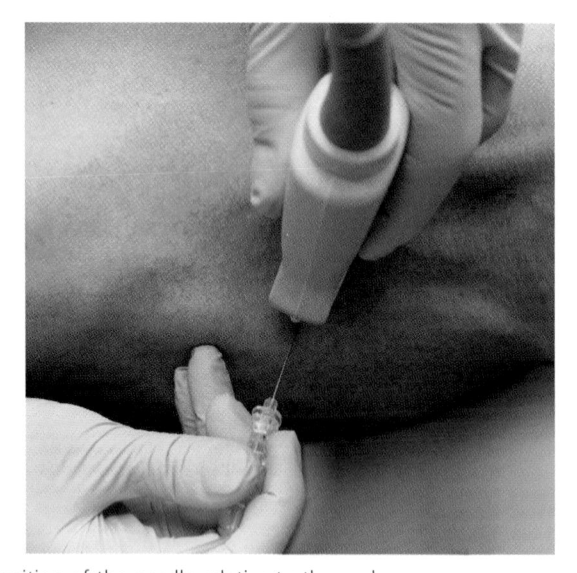

Fig. A4 IP position of the needle relative to the probe.

Training

- Basic knowledge in ultrasound physics and machine adjustment is required.
- Basic anatomy and sonoanatomy of the relevant areas of interest is mandatory.

- An understanding of needle guidance techniques, as described in 'Definitions,' is a prerequisite for a safe and successful performance of regional blocks.
- Start with level I blocks.

Ultrasound-guided nerve block rating scale

This is a classification of ultrasound-guided peripheral nerve blocks, ranging from level I (basic) to level III (advanced), based upon the following four criteria:

- Ease of visualization of nerve structures: 1 (easy), 2 (intermediate), 3 (difficult).
- Ease of visualization of identifying feature(s): 1 (easy), 2 (intermediate), 3 (difficult).
- Technical performance of block: 1 (easy), 2 (intermediate), 3 (difficult).
- Risk of complications from associated structures: 1 (low), 2 (intermediate), 3 (high).

- Level I blocks (basic): superficial cervical, interscalene, axillary, terminal branches of the brachial plexus (ulnar/median/radial)–forearm and arm, femoral, saphenous, ankle, ilioinguinal-iliohypogastric, rectus sheath.
- Level II blocks (intermediate): supraclavicular, infraclavicular, obturator (anterior and posterior branches), sciatic–posterior and lateral approaches (subgluteal, mid-femoral, and popliteal levels), sciatic–anterior approach, intercostals.
- Level III blocks (advanced): deep cervical, lumbar plexus (posterior approach), thoracic paravertebral.

Table 10 Summary score based on the 'Ultrasound-guided Nerve Block Rating Scale'

Summary score	Level	Description
4–6	I	Basic
7–9	II	Intermediate
10–12	III	Advanced

Sterility

- Protect the probe with a cover to minimize patient-patient disease transmission.
- An aseptic needle insertion technique is recommended.

Machine requirements

- Adequate software for small parts ultrasonography.
- Data storage (still and video).
- High-frequency probes are appropriate for superficial blocks.

Table 11 Definition of ultrasound probes

Definition of probe	Frequency
High frequency	>10MHz, linear
Medium frequency	6–10MHz, linear
Low frequency	2–5MHz, curved

Table 12 Particular peripheral regional anaesthetic techniques, probe recommendations, and levels of classification

Technique	Probe recommendation*	Summary score of 4 criteria (see above)**
Superficial cervical	High frequency, linear	6
Deep cervical	Medium frequency, linear	10
Interscalene	High frequency, linear	5
Supraclavicular	High frequency, linear	7
Infraclavicular	Medium frequency, linear	7
Axillary	High frequency, linear	6
Terminal branches of brachial plexus (ulnar/median/radial)–forearm and arm	High frequency, linear	5
Femoral	High frequency, linear	5
Saphenous	High frequency, linear	6
Obturator (anterior and posterior branches)	High frequency, linear	7
Sciatic (subgluteal, mid-femoral, and popliteal levels)–posterior and lateral approaches	Medium frequency, linear	7
Sciatic–anterior approach	Low frequency, curved	9
Ankle blocks	High frequency, linear	6
Lumbar plexus (posterior approach)	Low frequency, curved	11
Intercostal	High frequency, linear	8
Ilioinguinal-iliohypogastric	High frequency, linear	5
Rectus sheath	High frequency, linear	6
Thoracic paravertebral	Medium frequency, linear	10

* The recommendations are based on normal weight patients and may differ in obese patients; ** The summary score is the result of the mean evaluations of the 14 participants in the expert meeting.

Needles

The following needle properties are recommended:

- Short bevel needles to facilitate needle tip visibility, especially for OOP insertions.
- Needle length selection appropriate to the needle guidance technique (IP or OOP technique).
- Special echogenic needles show only minor advantage, mainly for IP technique.

A needle with its orifice at some distance from the needle tip (e.g. Whitacre spinal or Sprotte needles) is not recommended because of disproportion between the ultrasonographically visible tip of the needle and the real outflow of local anaesthetic.

Conclusions and future directions

An expert statement in a relatively new field of interest can only serve as a current opinion. Experience and evidenced knowledge in ultrasonographic guidance is limited in comparison to more established techniques of nerve identification during regional blocks. Therefore, it is clear that the experts' opinion may have to be adapted at regular intervals. Nevertheless, safe and effective blocks should be achieved by using expert opinion in terms of recommendations, training, sterility, and machine and needle requirements. This expert statement should also work as a basis for a future process of discussion and every user of these techniques is more than welcome to actively participate in future developments in order to raise ultrasound guidance in regional anaesthesia to an adequate level of evidence that finally a maximum number of patients benefit from the 'state of the art' techniques.

Appendix 2

Vienna score

Table 13 The Vienna score for ultrasonographic-guided nerve blocks

Score	Description
1	The internal structure of the nerve visualized
2	The nerve is visualized as a circular or oval bright hallo (epineurium)
3	The nerve is visualized as reflections determined by the anatomy of the surrounded tissue
4	The anatomical position of the nerve shows no response to the ultrasound beam (isoechoic behaviour)

Appendix 3

Guidelines for the management of severe local anaesthetic toxicity according to the Association of Anaesthetists of Great Britain and Ireland (2007)

Signs of severe toxicity

- Sudden loss of consciousness, with or without tonic-clonic convulsions.
- Cardiovascular collapse: sinus bradycardia, conduction blocks, asystole and ventricular tachyarrhythmia may all occur.
- Local anaesthetic toxicity may occur some time after the initial injection.

Immediate management

- Stop injecting the local anaesthetic.
- Call for help.
- Maintain the airway and, if necessary, secure it with a tracheal tube.
- Give 100% oxygen and ensure adequate lung ventilation (hyperventilation may help increase the pH in the presence of metabolic acidosis).
- Confirm or establish intravenous access.
- Control seizures: give a benzodiazepine, thiopental, or propofol in small incremental doses.
- Assess cardiovascular status throughout.

Management of cardiac arrest associated with local anaesthetic injection

- Start cardiopulmonary resuscitation (CPR) using standard protocols.
- Manage arrhythmias using the same protocols, recognizing that they may be very refractory to treatment.

- Prolonged resuscitation may be necessary; it may be appropriate to consider other options:
  - Consider the use of cardiopulmonary bypass if available.
  - Consider treatment with lipid emulsion.

Treatment of cardiac arrest with lipid emulsion

- Approximate doses are given in red for a 70kg patient.
- Give an intravenous bolus injection of Intralipid® 20%, 1.5mL/kg over 1min.
- Give a bolus of 100mL.
- Continue CPR.
- Start an intravenous infusion of Intralipid® 20% at a rate of 0.25mL/kg/min.
- Give at a rate of 400mL over 20min.
- Repeat the bolus injection twice at 5min intervals if an adequate circulation has not been restored.
- Give two further boluses of 100mL at 5min intervals.
- After another 5min, increase the rate to 0.5mL/kg/min if an adequate circulation has not been restored.
- Give at a rate of 400mL over 10min.
- Continue the infusion until a stable and adequate circulation has been restored.

Remember

- Continue CPR throughout the treatment with lipid emulsion.
- Recovery from local anaesthetic-induced cardiac arrest may take longer than 1h.
- Propofol is not a suitable substitute for Intralipid® 20%.
- Replace your supply of Intralipid® 20% after use.

Follow-up action

- Report cases to your national anaesthesia society.
- If possible, take blood samples into a plain tube and a heparinized tube before and after lipid emulsion administration and at 1h intervals afterwards. Ask your laboratory to measure local anaesthetic and triglyceride levels

(these have not yet been reported in a human case of local anaesthetic intoxication treated with lipid).

Notes

Intralipid® 20% has been shown to reverse local anaesthetic-induced cardiac arrest in animal models and in human case reports and its use has been reported in the treatment of life-threatening toxicity without cardiac arrest. Its therapeutic potential has been highlighted by the National Patient Safety Agency.

A total of 1000mL Intralipid® 20% should be immediately available in all areas where potentially cardiotoxic doses of local anaesthetics are given, along with guidelines for its use. Intralipid® is readily available from most hospital pharmacies, which may also be able to help departments with timely replacement of bags nearing expiry. The usefulness of other lipid emulsions is not known as published work to date has only used Intralipid®.

Although some propofol preparations are provided in Intralipid®, e.g. Diprivan®, these are not suitable alternatives due to a significant cardiovascular depression caused by propofol. This does not preclude the use of small, incremental doses of propofol to control seizures. The use of Intralipid® in this way is relatively novel. Therefore, future laboratory and clinical experiments are likely to dictate further refinement of the method.

This guideline document will be reviewed regularly and updated when necessary. Updated versions will be available on http://www.aagbi.org and http://www.lipidrescue.org. Further educational matter is available at http://www.lipidrescue.org. This guideline is not a standard of medical care. The ultimate judgement with regard to a particular clinical procedure or treatment plan must be made by the clinician in light of the clinical data presented and the diagnostic and treatment options available.

Suggested further reading

Foxall, G., McCahon, R., Lamb, J., Hardman, J.G., Bedforth, N.M., 2007. Levobupivacaine-induced seizures and cardiovascular collapse treated with Intralipid. *Anaesthesia*, 62(5), pp.516–8.

Litz, R.J., Popp, M., Stehr, S.N., Koch, T., 2006. Successful resuscitation of a patient with ropivacaine-induced asystole after axillary plexus block using lipid infusion. *Anaesthesia*, 61(8), pp.800–1.

National Patient Safety Agency, 28 March 2007. Patient safety alert 21–Safer practice with epidural injections and infusions. London. Available at: www.npsa.nhs.uk.

Rosenblatt, M.A., Abel, M., Fischer, G.W., Itzkovich, C.J., Eisenkraft, J.B., 2006. Successful use of a 20% lipid emulsion to resuscitate a patient after a presumed bupivacaine-related cardiac arrest. *Anesthesiology*, 105(1), pp.217–8.

Weinberg, G., Ripper, R., Feinstein, D.L., Hoffman, W., 2003. Lipid emulsion infusion rescues dogs from bupivacaine-induced cardiac toxicity. *Regional Anesthesia and Pain Medicine*, 28(3), pp.198–202.

Weinberg, G.L., VadeBoncouer, T., Ramaraju, G.A., Garcia–Amaro, M.F., Cwik, M.J., 1998. Pretreatment or resuscitation with a lipid infusion shifts the dose-response to bupivacaine-induced asystole in rats. *Anesthesiology*, 88(4), pp.1071–5.

Appendix 4

Definition of specific terms

Hyperechoic	Bright relative to the surrounding tissues
Hypoechoic	Dark relative to the surrounding tissues
Isoechoic	Equal relative to the surrounding tissues

Index

Note: Page numbers in *italics* indicate references to figures, pages numbers in **bold** indicate references to tables.

Q

R

S

T

U

V

W